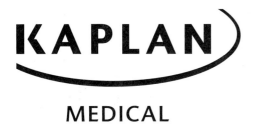

MEDICAL

USMLE®

STEP 2 CK

Lecture Notes 2017

Pediatrics

© 2016 by Kaplan, Inc.

Published by Kaplan Medical, a division of Kaplan, Inc.
750 Third Avenue
New York, NY 10017

10 9 8 7 6 5 4 3 2 1

Course ISBN: 978-1-5062-0805-3

Retail Kit ISBN: 978-1-5062-0816-9
This item comes as a set and should not be broken out and sold separately.

Kaplan Publishing print books are available at special quantity discounts to use for sales promotions, employee premiums, or educational purposes. For more information or to purchase books, please call the Simon & Schuster special sales department at 866-506-1949.

Editors

William G. Cvetnic, M.D., M.B.A.
Fellow of the American Academy of Pediatrics
Board Certified in Pediatrics and Neonatal-Perinatal Medicine
Jacksonville, Florida

Eduardo Pino, M.D.
Associate Professor, Department of Pediatrics
Marshall University School of Medicine
Medical Director, Pediatric ICU
Cabell Huntington Hospital
Huntington, West Virginia

We want to hear what you think. What do you like or not like about the Notes? Please email us at **medfeedback@kaplan.com**.

Contents

The Newborn

Learning Objectives

❏ Calculate an Apgar score

❏ Use knowledge of birth injuries to predict symptomology

❏ Demonstrate understanding of newborn screening, fetal growth/maturity, and neonatal infections

APGAR SCORE

A newborn infant at birth is noted to have acrocyanosis, heart rate 140/min, and grimaces to stimulation. She is active and has a lusty cry. What is her Apgar score?

Table 1-1. Apgar Scoring System

Evaluation	0 Points	1 Point	2 Points
Heart rate	0	<100/min	>100/min
Respiration	None	Irregular, shallow, gasps	Crying
Color	Blue	Pale, blue extremities	Pink
Tone	None	Weak, passive	Active
Reflex irritability	None	Facial grimace	Active withdrawal

Apgar scores are routinely assessed at 1 and 5 minutes, and every 5 minutes thereafter as long as resuscitation is continuing.

- The **1-minute score** gives an idea of what was going on during labor and delivery.
- The **5-minute score** gives an idea of response to therapy (resuscitation).

In general, the Apgar score is *not* predictive of outcome; however, infants with score 0–3 at ≥5 minutes compared to infants with score 7–10 have a worse neurologic outcome.

KAPLAN) MEDICAL   1

Newborn Care

- Vitamin K IM
- Prophylactic eye erythromycin
- Umbilical cord care
- Hearing test
- Newborn screening tests

BIRTH INJURIES

On physical exam, a 12-h-old newborn is noted to have nontender swelling of the head that does not cross the suture line. What is the most likely diagnosis?

Table 1-2. Common Injuries During Deliveries

Injury	Specifics	Outcome
Skull fractures	In utero from pressure against bones or forceps; **linear:** most common	• Linear: no symptoms and no treatment needed • **Depressed:** elevate to prevent cortical injury
Brachial palsy	**Erb-Duchenne:** C5–C6; cannot abduct shoulder; externally rotate and supinate forearm; **Klumpke:** C7–C8 ± T1; paralyzed hand ± Horner syndrome	Most with full recovery (months); depends on whether nerve was injured or lacerated; Rx: proper positioning and partial immobilization; massage and range of motion exercises; if no recovery in 3–6 mo, then neuroplasty
Clavicular fracture	Especially with shoulder dystocia in vertex position and arm extension in breech	Palpable callus within a week; Rx: with immobilization of arm and shoulder
Facial nerve palsy	Entire side of face with forehead; forceps delivery or in utero pressure over facial nerve	Improvement over weeks (as long as fibers were not torn); need eye care; neuroplasty if no improvement (torn fibers)
Caput succedaneum	Diffuse edematous swelling of soft tissues of scalp; **crosses suture lines**	Disappears in first few days; may lead to molding for weeks
Cephalohematoma	Subperiosteal hemorrhage: **does not cross suture lines**	May have underlying linear fracture; resolve in 2 wk to 3 mo; may calcify; jaundice

KAPLAN) MEDICAL

PHYSICAL EXAMINATION—NORMAL AND ABNORMAL FINDINGS

A newborn infant has a blue-gray pigmented lesion on the sacral area. It is clearly demarcated and does not fade into the surrounding skin. What is the most likely diagnosis?

A newborn has a flat, salmon-colored lesion on the glabella, which becomes darker red when he cries. What is the best course of management?

Table 1-3. Physical Examination—Common Findings (*see* remaining chapter for other specific findings)

Finding/Diagnosis	Description/Comments
SKIN	
Cutis marmorata	Lacy, reticulated vascular pattern over most of body when baby is cooled; improves over first month; abnormal if persists
Salmon patch (nevus simplex)	Pale, pink vascular macules; found in nuchal area, glabella, eyelids; usually disappears
Mongolian spots	Blue to slate-gray macules; seen on presacral, back, posterior thighs; > in nonwhite infants; arrested melanocytes; usually fade over first few years; *differential*: child abuse
Erythema toxicum, neonatorum	Firm, yellow-white papules/pustules with erythematous base; peaks on second day of life; contain eosinophils; benign
Hemangioma	**Superficial**: bright red, protuberant, sharply demarcated; most often appear in first 2 months; most on face, scalp, back, anterior chest; rapid expansion, then stationary, then involution (most by 5–9 years of age); **deeper**: bluish hue, firm, cystic, less likely to regress; Rx: (steroids, pulsed laser) only if large and interfering with function
HEAD	
Preauricular tags/pits	Look for hearing loss and genitourinary anomalies.
Coloboma of iris	Cleft at "six o'clock" position; most with other eye abnormalities; CHARGE association
Aniridia	Hypoplasia of iris; defect may go through to retina; association with Wilms tumor
EXTREMITIES	
Polydactyly	>5 number of fingers or toes. No treatment needed if good blood supply.

NEWBORN SCREENING

A 1-month-old fair-haired, fair-skinned baby presents with projectile vomiting of 4 days' duration. Physical exam reveals a baby with eczema and a musty odor. Which screening test would most likely be abnormal?

Every newborn is screened before discharge or day 4 of life. It is more reliable if done after 48 hours of oral feedings (substrates for metabolic diseases).

The total diseases screened are determined by the individual state. Some examples:

- Phenylketonuria
- Tyrosinemia
- 21-hydroxylase deficiency
- Galactosemia
- Hb SS
- Hb C
- Hypothyroidism
- Cystic fibrosis

Table 1-4. Comparison of Two Newborn Screening Diseases*

	Phenylketonuria (PKU)	**Classic Galactosemia**
Defect	Phenylalanine hydroxylase; accumulation of PHE in body fluids and CNS	Gal-1-P uridylyltransferase deficiency; accumulation of gal-1-P with injury to **kidney, liver, and brain**
Presentation	**Mental retardation,** vomiting, growth retardation, purposeless movements, athetosis, seizures	**Jaundice (often direct),** hepatomegaly, vomiting, **hypoglycemia, cataracts,** seizures, poor feeding, poor weight gain, **mental retardation**
Associations	**Fair hair, fair skin, blue eyes,** tooth abnormalities, microcephaly	**Predisposition to *E. coli* sepsis;** developmental delay, speech disorders, learning disabilities
Other comments	**Normal at birth;** gradual MR over first few months	**May begin prenatally— transplacental galactose from mother**
Treatment	Low PHE diet for life	No lactose—reverses growth failure, kidney and liver abnormalities and cataracts, **but not neurodevelopmental problems**

Definition of abbreviations: CNS, central nervous system; G-1-P, galactose-1-phosphate; MR, mental retardation; PHE, phenylalanine.
*Items in **bold** have a greater likelihood of appearing on the exam.

FETAL GROWTH AND MATURITY

Table 1-5. Intrauterine Growth Restriction (IUGR)

Type	Reason	Main Etiologies	Complications
Symmetric	Early, in utero insult that affects growth of most organs	Genetic syndromes, chromosomal abnormalities, congenital infections, teratogens, toxins	Etiology dependent; delivery of oxygen and nutrients to vital organs usually normal
Asymmetric (head sparing)	Relatively late onset after fetal organ development; abnormal delivery of nutritional substances and oxygen to the fetus	Uteroplacental insufficiency secondary to maternal diseases (malnutrition, cardiac, renal, anemia) and/or placental dysfunction (hypertension, autoimmune disease, abruption)	Neurologic (asphyxia) if significant decreased delivery of oxygen to brain

Gestational Age and Size at Birth		
Preterm	Large for Gestational Age (LGA)—Fetal Macrosomia	Post-term
• Premature—liveborn infants delivered prior to 37 weeks as measured from the first day of the last menstrual period • Low birth weight—birthweight <2,500 grams. This may be due to prematurity, IUGR, or both	• Birth weight >4,500 grams at term • Predisposing factors: obesity, diabetes • Higher incidence of birth injuries and congenital anomalies	• Infants born after 42 weeks' gestation from last menstrual period • **When delivery is delayed ≥3 weeks past term, significant increase in mortality.** • Characteristics 　– Increased birth weight 　– Absence of lanugo 　– Decreased/absent vernix 　– Desquamating, pale, loose skin 　– Abundant hair, long nails 　– If placental insufficiency, may be meconium staining

SPECIFIC DISORDERS

Endocrine Disorders

Infants of diabetic mothers

You are called to see a 9.5-pound newborn infant who is jittery. Physical exam reveals a large plethoric infant who is tremulous. A murmur is heard. Blood sugar is low.

- Maternal hyperglycemia (types I and II DM) → fetal hyperinsulinemia
- Insulin is the major fetal growth hormone → increase in size of all organs except the brain
- Major metabolic effect is at birth with sudden placental separation → **hypoglycemia**
- Infants may be **large for gestational age and plethoric** (ruddy).
- Other **metabolic findings: hypoglycemia and hypomagnesemia** (felt to be a result of delayed action of parathyroid hormone)
- **Common findings**
  - **Birth trauma** (macrosomia)
  - **Tachypnea** (transient tachypnea, respiratory distress syndrome, cardiac failure, hypoglycemia)
  - **Cardiomegaly—asymmetric septal hypertrophy** (insulin effect, reversible)
  - **Polycythemia (and hyperviscosity)** → hyperbilirubinemia → jaundice
  - **Renal vein thrombosis** (flank mass, hematuria, and thrombocytopenia) from polycythemia
  - **Increased incidence of congenital anomalies**
    - **Cardiac**—especially VSD, ASD, transposition
    - **Small left colon syndrome** (transient delay in development of left side of colon; presents with abdominal distention)
    - **Caudal regression syndrome:** spectrum of structural neurologic defects of the caudal region of spinal cord which may result in neurologic impairment (hypo, aplasia of pelvis & LE)
- Prognosis—Infants of diabetic mothers are more predisposed to diabetes and LGA infants are at increased risk of childhood obesity.
- Treatment
  - Monitor carefully and advocate good glucose control during pregnancy. Follow glucose carefully in infant after delivery.
  - Early, frequent feeds: oral, NG if episodes of hypoglycemia continue
  - Intravenous dextrose infusion if above does not result in euglycemia

Respiratory Disorders

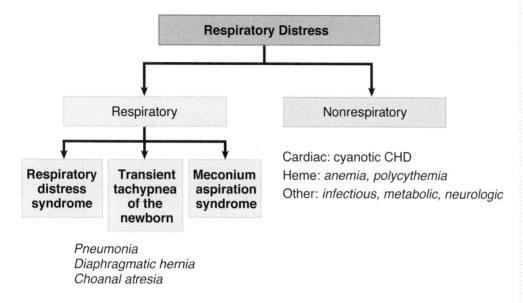

Figure 1-1. Respiratory Distress

Respiratory distress syndrome (RDS)

> Shortly after birth, a 33-week gestation infant develops tachypnea, nasal flaring, and grunting and requires intubation. Chest radiograph shows a hazy, ground-glass appearance of the lungs.

- Deficiency of **mature surfactant** (surfactant matures biochemically over gestation; therefore, the incidence of surfactant deficiency diminishes toward term.)

- Inability to maintain alveolar volume at end expiration → decreased FRC (functional residual capacity) and atelectasis

- Primary initial pulmonary hallmark is **hypoxemia.** Then, **hypercarbia and respiratory acidosis ensue.**

- Diagnosis
  - **Best initial diagnostic test—chest radiograph**
    - Findings: **ground-glass appearance, atelectasis, air bronchograms**
  - **Most accurate diagnostic test—L/S ratio** (part of complete lung profile; lecithin-to-sphingomyelin ratio)
    - Done on amniotic fluid prior to birth
  - **Best initial treatment—oxygen**
  - **Most effective treatment—intubation and exogenous surfactant administration**
  - **Primary prevention**
    - Avoid prematurity (tocolytics)
    - **Antenatal betamethasone**

Transient tachypnea of the newborn (TTN)

- Slow absorption of fetal lung fluid → decreased pulmonary compliance and tidal volume with increased dead space

- Tachypnea after birth

- Generally minimal oxygen requirement

- **Common in term infant delivered by Cesarean section or rapid second stage of labor**

- **Chest x-ray (best test)**—air-trapping, fluid in fissures, perihilar streaking

- Rapid improvement generally within hours to a few days

Meconium aspiration

- Meconium passed as a result of hypoxia and fetal distress; may be aspirated in utero or with the first postnatal breath → airway obstruction and pneumonitis → failure and pulmonary hypertension

- **Chest x-ray (best test)—patchy infiltrates, increased AP diameter, flattening of diaphragm**

- Other complications—air leak (pneumothorax, pneumomediastinum)

- **Prevention—endotracheal intubation and airway suction of depressed infants with thick meconium**

- Treatment—positive pressure ventilation and other complex NICU therapies

Diaphragmatic hernia

- Failure of the diaphragm to close → abdominal contents enter into chest, causing **pulmonary hypoplasia.**

- Born with respiratory distress and **scaphoid abdomen**

- **Bowel sounds may be heard in chest**

- Diagnosis—prenatal ultrasound; **postnatal x-ray (best test) reveals bowel in chest**

- Best initial treatment—immediate intubation in delivery room for known or suspected CDH, followed by surgical correction when stable (usually days)

Gastrointestinal and Hepatobiliary Disorders

See also GI chapter on this topic.

Umbilical hernia

- Failure of the umbilical ring closure, weakness of abdominal muscles

- Most are small and resolve in 1-2 years without any treatment

- Surgery if getting larger after 1-2 years, symptoms (strangulation, incarceration), and/or persistent after age 4

Omphalocele

- Failure of intestines to return to abdominal cavity with gut through umbilicus

- Covered in a sac (protection)

- Associated with other major malformations and possible genetic disorders (trisomy)

- Large defects need a staged reduction (use of a surgical Silo), otherwise respiratory failure and ischemia

Gastroschisis

- Defect in abdominal wall lateral to umbilicus (vascular accident)

- Any part of the GI tract may protrude

- Not covered by a sac

- Major problem with the intestines: atresia, stenosis, ischemia, short gut

- Surgery based on condition of gut; if no ischemia, large lesions need a staged reduction as with omphalocele

Necrotizing enterocolitis (NEC)

- Transmural intestinal necrosis

- Greatest risk factor is prematurity; rare in term infants

- Symptoms usually related to **introduction of feeds**: bloody stools, apnea, lethargy, and abdominal distention once perforation has occurred

- **Pneumatosis intestinalis** on plain abdominal film is pathognomonic (air in bowel wall)

- Treatment: cessation of feeds, gut decompression, systemic antibiotics, and supportive care; surgical resection of necrotic bowel may be necessary

Imperforate Anus

- Failure to pass stool after birth

- No anal opening visible

- Treatment is surgical correction.

- May be part of VACTERL association.

Jaundice

> A 2-day-old infant is noticed to be jaundiced. He is nursing and stooling well. Indirect bilirubin is 11.2 mg/dL; direct is 0.4 mg/dL. Physical exam is unremarkable except for visible jaundice.

- Pathophysiology
  - Increased production of bilirubin from breakdown of fetal red blood cells plus immaturity of hepatic conjugation of bilirubin and elimination in first week of life

– Rapidly increasing unconjugated (indirect reacting) bilirubin can cross the blood-brain barrier and lead to **kernicterus (unconjugated bilirubin in the basal ganglia and brain stem nuclei)** hypotonia, seizures, opisthotonos, delayed motor skills, choreoathetosis, and **sensorineural hearing loss** are features of kernicterus.

Table 1-6. Physiologic Jaundice Versus Pathologic Jaundice

Physiologic Jaundice	Pathologic Jaundice
Appears on second to third day of life (term)	May appear in first 24 hours of life
Disappears by fifth day of life (term)—7th	Variable
Peaks at second to third day of life	Variable
Peak bilirubin <13 mg/dL (term)	Unlimited
Rate of bilirubin rise <5 mg/dL/d	Usually >5 mg/dL/d

The **causes of hyperbilirubinemia** with respect to **bilirubin metabolism** are as follows:

• RBC metabolism

  – Increased number of RBCs

    ◦ Normal newborn (normal Hct is 42–65)

      i. Physiologic jaundice

    ◦ Polycythemia (Hct >65)

      i. **Increased RBC production:** Chronic hypoxia, IUGR, post-mature; IODM, Beckwith-Wiedemann syndrome (insulin effect); maternal Graves' disease (transplacental antibodies); trisomies (? mechanism)

      ii. **Extra RBCs entering the circulation:** delayed cord clamping, twin-twin transfusion, maternal-fetal transfusion

      iii. Treatment: partial exchange transfusion with normal saline (dilutional)

  – Increased hemolysis

    ◦ **Immune-mediated** (labs: high unconjugated bilirubin, may be anemia, increased reticulocyte count, **positive direct Coombs test**)

      i. Rh negative mother/Rh positive baby: classic hemolytic disease of the newborn (erythroblastosis fetalis)

      ii. ABO incompatibility (almost all are type O mother and either type A or B baby): most common reason for hemolysis in the newborn

      iii. Minor blood group incompatibility (Kell is very antigenic; Kell negative mother), uncommon

    ◦ **Non-immune mediated:** same as above but Coombs is negative; need to see blood smear

      i. Smear shows **characteristic-looking RBCs**: membrane defect (most are either spherocytosis or elliptocytosis)

ii. Smear shows **normal-looking RBCs**: enzyme defect (most are G6PD deficiency then pyruvate kinase deficiency)

iii. Extravascular: excessive bruising, cephalohematoma

- Bilirubin is then bound to albumin and carried in the blood; bilirubin may be uncoupled from albumin in the blood stream to yield free bilirubin, e.g. neonatal sepsis, certain drugs (ceftriaxone), hypoxia, acidosis.

- Bilirubin is transported to the hepatocytes: within the hepatocytes is the conversion of unconjugated (laboratory indirect-acting) fat-soluble bilirubin to conjugated (glucuronide) water-soluble bilirubin (laboratory direct-acting) by the action of **hepatic glucuronyl transferase (GT).**

  - Decreased enzymatic activity of GT

    ○ Normal newborn first week of life

    ○ Primary liver disease of systemic disease affecting the liver (sepsis, TORCH, metabolic diseases)

    ○ No GT activity: Crigler-Najjar syndrome (type I)

- Transport through the intrahepatic biliary system to the porta hepatis for excretion into the duodenum; abnormalities of transport and excretion cause a conjugated (direct) hyperbilirubinemia (**>2 mg/dL direct-acting bilirubin in the blood in the newborn**).

  - **Biliary atresia** (progressive obliterative cholangiopathy): obstruction at birth due to fibrosis and atresia of the extrahepatic ducts (and so no gall bladder); then variable severity and speed of inflammation and fibrosis of the intrahepatic system which ultimately leads to cirrhosis

    ○ Most present in first 2 weeks of life with jaundice (conjugated hyperbilirubinemia), poor feeding, vomiting, lethargy, hepatosplenomegaly, **persistent acholic stools and dark urine**

    ○ **Best initial test:** U/S (triangular fibrotic cord at porta hepatis; no evidence of normal ductal anatomy; no gallbladder

    ○ **Most accurate test** (next step): percutaneous liver biopsy (is pathognomonic for this process)

    ○ **Best initial treatment** (palliative): hepatic portojejunostomy (Kasai procedure)

    ○ **Best long-term management:** liver transplant

  - Liver disease (primary or secondary to systemic disease): cholestasis (sepsis, perinatal infections, metabolic disease, neonatal hepatitis, severe hypothyroidism and others

- Intestinal transport and excretion: most bilirubin is eliminated in the stool with final products synthesized with help of colonic bacteria; some bilirubin is eliminated in the urine, some is reprocessed in the liver due to enterohepatic circulation (along with bile acids); **intestinal beta-glucuronidase** hydrolyzes glucuronide-bilirubin bonds to yield some unconjugated bilirubin, which is absorbed into the portal circulation and transported back to the liver to be acted upon by hepatic glucuronyl transferase

  - **Increased enterohepatic circulation**

    ○ Intestinal obstruction

    ○ Decreased colonic bacteria (first week of life, prolonged antibiotics, severe diarrhea)

Breast feeding jaundice vs. breast milk jaundice (see text box)

```
                  ┌──────────────┐          ┌──────────────┐
                  │  Physiologic │──────────│  Pathologic  │
                  └──────────────┘          └──────────────┘
                         │                         │
                  ┌──────────────┐                 │
                  │   Indirect   │◄────────────────┘
                  └──────────────┘
```

Direct
- Sepsis
- TORCH infections
- Hypothyroidism
- Galactosemia
- Cystic fibrosis
- Choledochal cyst
- Biliary atresia
- Dubin-Johnson
- Rotor syndrome

Coombs (+)
- Rh/ABO incompatibility
- Minor blood groups

Coombs (–)

High Hgb
- Polycythemia
  - Twin-twin transfusion
  - Maternal-fetal transfusion
  - Delayed cord
  - IUGR
  - Infant of diabetic mother

Normal/low Hgb
- Spherocytosis
- Elliptocytosis
- G6PD deficiency
- Pyruvate kinase
- Hemorrhage
- Cephalohematoma bruising
- Bowel obstruction
- Breast feeding
- Crigler-Najjar
- Gilbert syndrome

Figure 1-2. Jaundice Workup

Breast-Feeding Jaundice versus Breast-Milk Jaundice

Breast-feeding jaundice means a baby is not nursing well and so not getting many calories. This is common in first-time breast-feeding mothers. The infant may become dehydrated; however, it is lack of calories that causes the jaundice. Treatment is to obtain a lactation consultation and rehydrate the baby. The jaundice occurs in the first days of life.

Breast-milk jaundice occurs due to a glucoronidase present in some breast milk. Infants become jaundiced in week 2 of life. Treatment is phototherapy if needed. Although the bilirubin may rise again, it will not rise to the previous level. The baby may then be safely breast fed. The jaundice will be gone by 2–3 months.

- Treatment of hyperbilirubinemia
  - Phototherapy
    - Complications: loose stools, erythematous macular rash, overheating leading to dehydration, and **bronze baby syndrome (occurs with direct hyperbilirubinemia; dark, grayish-brown discoloration of the skin** [photo-induced change in porphyrins, which are present in cholestatic jaundice])
  - Double volume exchange transfusion—if bilirubin continues to rise despite intensive phototherapy and/or kernicterus is a concern

Table 1-7. Hyperbilirubinemia and Jaundice

Etiology	Reason for increased bilirubin	Hyperbilirubinemia	Hgb, Hct/ Reticulocytes	Other labs	Treatment
Excessive bruising/ cephalohematoma	RBCs → Hgb → Bilirubin	Indirect	• Normal to slightly low Hgb/Hct • Normal to slight increase in reticulocytes		Phototherapy
Immune hemolysis • Rh • ABO • Minor blood groups	Anti-Rh, anti-A, anti-B, anti-minor blood group Abs	Indirect	• Low Hgb/Hct (anemia) • Increased reticulocytes	• Rh negative mother and Rh positive baby • Type O mother and type A or B baby • Direct Coombs positive • Decreased RBCs	Phototherapy + possible exchange transfusion
Polycythemia	High Hct, Hgb → high bilirubin	Indirect	High (Hct >65)/ normal	Increased RBCs	Phototherapy + partial exchange transfusion
Non-immune hemolysis	Abnormal RBC → splenic removal	Indirect	Low (anemia)/ increased	• If no membrane defect →, G6PD, PK activity • Characteristic RBCs if membrane defect • Decreased RBCs	Phototherapy + transfusion
Displacement of bound bilirubin from albumin	Free bilirubin in circulation	Indirect	Normal		Treat underlying problem
Familial nonhemolytic hyperbilirubinemia (Crigler-Najjar syndrome)	Absence of glucuronyl transferase (type I) vs. small amount of inducible GT (type II)	Indirect	Normal	GT activity	Phototherapy + exchange transfusion
Extrahepatic obstruction— biliary atresia	Bilirubin cannot leave the biliary system	Direct	Normal	Ultrasound, liver biopsy	Portojejunostomy, then later liver transplant
Cholestasis (TORCH, sepsis, metabolic, endocrine)	Abnormal hepatic function → decrease bilirubin excretion	Direct	Normal	With H and P, other select labs suggestive of underlying etiology	Treat underlying problem
Bowel obstruction	Increased enterohepatic recirculation	Indirect	Normal		Relieve obstruction + phototherapy
Breast feeding jaundice	Increased enterohepatic recirculation	Indirect	Normal		Phototherapy + hydration + teach breast feeding
Breast milk jaundice	Increased enterohepatic,, recirculation	Indirect	Normal		Phototherapy + continued breast feeding

INFECTIONS

Neonatal Sepsis

A 3-week-old infant presents with irritability, poor feeding, temperature of 38.9°C (102°F), and grunting. Physical examination reveals a bulging fontanel, delayed capillary refill, and grunting.

- Signs and symptoms are very nonspecific.
- Risk factors
    - Prematurity
    - Chorioamnionitis
    - Intrapartum fever
    - Prolonged rupture of membranes
- **Most common organisms: group B *Streptococcus*, *E. coli*, and *Listeria monocytogenes*.**
- **Diagnosis**—sepsis workup: CBC, differential and platelets, blood culture, urine analysis and culture, chest radiograph (Lumbar puncture not routinely performed unless there is a likelihood of meningitis, e.g., irritability, lethargy, hypothermia, etc.)
- **Treatment**
    - **If no evidence of meningitis: ampicillin and aminoglycoside until 48–72-hour cultures are negative**
    - **If meningitis or diagnosis is possible: ampicillin and third-generation cephalosporin (*not* ceftriaxone)**

Transplacental Intrauterine Infections (TORCH)

TORCH infections are typically acquired in first or second trimester. Most infants have IUGR.

Toxoplasmosis

Toxoplasmosis is a maternal infection worldwide, due primarily to ingestion of undercooked or raw meat containing tissue cysts. Ingestion of water or food with oocytes that have been excreted by infected cats (fecal contamination) is the most common form of transmission in the United States. Advise pregnant women not to change/clean cat litter while pregnant.

- Findings
    - Jaundice, hepatosplenomegaly
    - Thrombocytopenia, anemia
    - Microcephaly
    - **Chorioretinitis**
    - **Hydrocephalus**
    - **Intracranial calcifications**
    - Seizures

Note

Toxoplasmosis

Other (syphilis, varicella, HIV, and parvovirus B19)

Rubella

Cytomegalovirus (CMV)

Herpes

- Outcomes
  - Psychomotor retardation
  - Seizure disorder
  - **Visual impairments**
- **Treatment—maternal treatment during pregnancy reduces the likelihood of transmission significantly (spiramycin)**
  - Infants are treated with pyrimethamine, sulfadiazine, and leucovorin.

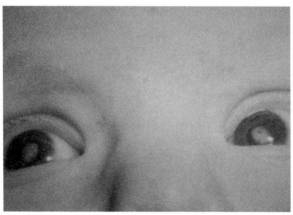

phil.cdc.gov

Figure 1-3. Congenital Cataract Secondary to Maternal Rubella Infection

Congenital rubella

- Classic findings when maternal infection occurs in first 8 weeks' gestation.
- Findings
  - **Blueberry muffin spots** (extramedullary hematopoiesis), thrombocytopenia
  - Cardiac—**PDA, peripheral pulmonary artery stenosis**
  - Eye—**cataracts**
  - **Congenital hearing loss**
  - Thrombocytopenia
  - Hepatosplenomegaly
- Outcomes
  - Hearing loss
  - Persistent growth retardation
  - Microcephaly
  - Mental and motor retardation

Cytomegalovirus (CMV)

- Primary infection (higher risk of severe disease) or reactivation of CMV
- Findings
  - Hepatosplenomegaly, jaundice
  - **Periventricular calcifications**
  - **Intrauterine growth retardation**

- Chorioretinitis
- **Microcephaly**
- Thrombocytopenia, hemolytic anemia
- Outcomes
  - **Sensorineural hearing loss**
  - Neuromuscular abnormalities
  - **Mental retardation**

Herpes simplex

- Keratojunctivitis, skin (5–14 days), CNS (3–4 weeks), disseminated (5–7 days)
- Best diagnosis: PCR, any body fluid
- Best treatment: IV acyclovir ASAP
- Outcomes
  - Microcephaly, spasticity
  - Deafness
  - Blindness
  - Seizure disorder
  - Psychomotor retardation
  - Death
- **Prevention is elective Cesarean section when active disease or visible lesions are identified; however, this is not 100% effective.**
- **Treatment—acyclovir**

Congenital syphilis

- Transplacental transmission usually during second half of gestation
- **At-risk infants must undergo serologic testing at the time of delivery.**
- Findings
  - Early (birth–2 yrs): snuffles, maculopapular rash (including palms of soles, desquamates), jaundice, periostitis, osteochondritis, chorioretinitis, congenital nephrosis
  - Late (>2 years of age): Hutchinson teeth, Clutton joints, saber shins, saddle nose, osteochondritis, rhagades (thickening and fissures of corners of mouth)
- **Diagnosis—*Treponema* in scrapings (most accurate test) from any lesion or fluid, serologic tests**
  - Infant with positive VDRL plus pathognomonic signs; if not, perform serial determinations—increasing titer in infection
  - **Most helpful specific test is IgM-FTA-ABS (immunoglobin fluorescent treponemal antibody absorption); but it is not always positive immediately.**
- **Treatment—penicillin**

Varicella

- Neonatal
  - Seen when delivery occurs <1 week before/after maternal infection
  - Treat with VZIG (varicella zoster immune globulin), if mother develops varicella 5 days before to 2 days after delivery.

- Congenital
    - Associated with limb malformations and deformations, cutaneous scars, microcephaly, chorioretinitis, cataracts, and cortical atrophy
    - Associated with infection during 1st or 2nd trimester

Many of the findings of the **TORCH infections** are very similar, so note the most likely presentations:

- Toxoplasmosis: hydrocephalus with **generalized calcifications** and chorioretinitis
- Rubella: the classic findings of **cataracts, deafness, and heart defects**
- CMV: microcephaly with **periventricular calcifications**; petechiae with thrombocytopenia
- Herpes: skin vesicles, keratoconjunctivitis, acute meningoencephalitis
- Syphilis: osteochondritis and periostitis; skin rash involving palms and soles and is desquamating; **snuffles** (mucopurulent rhinitis)

SUBSTANCE ABUSE AND NEONATAL WITHDRAWAL

A 2-day-old infant is noticed to have coarse jitters and is very irritable with a high-pitched cry. A low-grade fever is reported, as well as diarrhea. Maternal history is positive for heroin use.

Table 1-8. Neonatal Features of Maternal Major Illicit Drug Use

Opiates	Cocaine
High incidence low birth weight, most with intrauterine growth restriction	No classic withdrawal symptoms
Increased rate of stillborns	Preterm labor, abruption, asphyxia
No increase in congenital abnormalities	Intrauterine growth restriction
Early withdrawal symptoms, within 48 hours	Impaired auditory processing, developmental delay, learning disabilities
Tremors and hyperirritability	High degree of polysubstance abuse
Diarrhea, apnea, poor feeding, high-pitched cry, weak suck, weight loss, tachypnea, hyperacusis, seizures, others	Central nervous system ischemic and hemorrhagic lesions
Increased risk of sudden infant death syndrome	Vasoconstriction → other malformations

- Diagnostic tests: a good history and the clinical presentation usually are sufficient to make the diagnosis. Meconium toxicology can detect opioid and cocaine exposure after the first trimester. Urine drug screening provides maternal drug use data for only a few days prior to delivery. Cord blood sample has become the best test for diagnosis.

- Treatment: narcotics, sedatives, and hypnotics, as well as swaddling and reducing noxious stimulation

- Complications: infants of addicted mothers are at higher risk for low birth weight, IUGR, congenital anomalies (alcohol, cocaine), and sudden infant death syndrome, as well as of mother's complications, such as sexually transmitted diseases, toxemia, breech, abruption, and intraventricular hemorrhage (cocaine).

Genetics/Dysmorphology 2

Learning Objectives

❏ Demonstrate understanding of chromosome abnormalities

❏ Solve problems concerning early overgrowth with associated defects, defects with facial features as the major defect, osteochondrodysplasias, and disorders of connective tissue

❏ Explain information related to unusual brain and/or neuromuscular findings with associated defects

ABNORMALITIES OF CHROMOSOMES

Trisomy 21 (Down Syndrome)

Down syndrome is the **most common** pattern of human malformation.

- Genetics
  - 94% full trisomy 21(nondisjunction); risk of recurrence 1–2% and then increases with **advancing maternal age**
  - 4–6% with translocation; most are new mutations but must obtain parental karyotypes for possible balanced translocation carrier
- Findings
  - **Upward slanting palpebral fissures; speckling of iris (Brushfield spots); inner epicanthal folds**
  - Small stature, mouth open with tongue protrusion; mild microcephaly, short neck, flat occiput, short metacarpals and phalanges; **single palmar crease**
  - **Hypotonia**
  - **Hearing loss (sensorineural, conductive, and mixed)**
  - Primary gonadal deficiency
  - **Cardiac anomaly—ECD > VSD > PDA, ASD; also MVP**
  - Gastrointestinal anomalies: **duodenal atresia, Hirschprung**
  - **Atlanto-axial instability**
  - **Hypothyroidism**
  - **Acute lymphocytic leukemia** (but acute myeloblastic leukemia if in first 3 years of life)
  - **Mental retardation, variable**

Cardiac Abbreviations

ASD: atrial septal defect

ECD: endocardial cushion defect

MVP: mitral valve prolapse

PDA: patent ductus arteriosus

TOF: tetralogy of Fallot

VSD: ventricular septal defect

- Natural history
  - Major cause for early mortality is congenital heart disease
  - Muscle tone improves with age
  - Rate of development slows with age
  - Early onset of Alzheimer disease

Trisomy 18 (Edwards Syndrome)

Edwards syndrome is the **second most common** pattern of human malformation.

- Genetics—older maternal age; nondisjunction
- Findings
  - Growth deficiency
  - **Mental retardation**
  - **Low-set, malformed ears; microcephaly, micrognathia; prominent occiput**
  - **Clenched hand—index over third; fifth over fourth**
  - **Short sternum**
  - **VSD, ASD, PDA, cyanotic lesions,**
  - **Rocker-bottom feet, hammer toe**
  - **Omphalocele**
- Natural history
  - Many spontaneous abortions
  - Feeble from birth
  - Most do not survive first year

Trisomy 13 (Patau Syndrome)

Patau syndrome is a defect of midface, eye, and forebrain development → single defect in first 3 weeks' development of prechordal mesoderm. It involves older maternal age.

- Findings
  - **Holoprosencephaly and other CNS defects**
  - **Severe mental retardation**
  - **Microcephaly; microphthalmia**
  - **Severe cleft lip, palate, or both**
  - **Scalp defects in parietal-occipital area** (cutis aplasia)
  - **Postaxial polydactyly**
  - VSD, PDA, ASD, cyanotic lesions
  - Single umbilical artery

Aniridia–Wilms Tumor Association (WAGR Syndrome)

- Genetics
  - 1/70 with aniridia also has Wilms
  - WAGR syndrome: deletion of 11p13; **W**ilms + **A**niridia + **G**U anomalies + M**R**
  - Highest risk of Wilms' (compared to independent aniridia or GU defect)

Klinefelter Syndrome (XXY)

- Genetics; most common findings manifested at puberty
- Findings
  - **Decreased IQ** (average IQ 85–90)
  - **Behavioral/psychiatric problems**
  - **Long limbs** (decreased upper:lower segment ratio)
  - Slim (weight/height ratio low)
  - **Hypogonadism and hypogenitalism** (testosterone replacement at age 11–12 years) = hypergonadotrophic hypogonadism (increased FSH and LH, and decreased testosterone)
  - Infertilty in almost all
  - Gynecomastia

Turner Syndrome (XO)

- Genetics
  - Generally sporadic; no older maternal age seen
  - Paternal chromosome more likely to be missing
  - Many mosiac patterns (including Y-chromatin)
- Findings
  - Small-stature female
  - Gonadal dysgenesis–streak ovaries in XO
  - Average IQ 90
  - **Congenital lymphedema, residual puffiness over dorsum of fingers and toes**
  - **Broad chest, wide-spaced nipples**
  - **Low posterior hairline; webbed posterior neck**
  - **Cubitus valgus (elbow) and other joint problems**
  - **Horseshoe kidney, and other renal defects**
  - Cardiac:
    - **Bicuspid aortic valve** (number 1 cardiac anomaly)
    - **Coarctation**
    - Aortic stenosis, mitral valve prolapse
    - Hypertension common, even without cardiac or renal disease
  - Primary hypothyroidism, mostly autoimmune, and other autoimmune diseases (celiac disease)
- Natural history
  - Decreased height velocity with delayed bone age
  - **Estrogen treatment indicated**
  - **May increase height by 3–4 cm with growth hormone (GH)**

Note

Gonadal dysgenesis is not evident in childhood, so chromosomes are warranted in any short-stature female whose phenotype is compatible with Turner syndrome.

Also consider in any adolescent with absent breast development by age 13, pubertal arrest, or primary/secondary amenorrhea with increased FSH.

Fragile X Syndrome

- Genetics
  - Fragile site on long arm of X in affected males and some carrier females—Molecular diagnosis—variable number of repeat CGG (preferred diagnosis = DNA-based molecular analysis)
  - X-linked dominant—males (most common cause of inherited mental retardation); girls have lower number of trinucleotide sequences → NL phenotype but may have lower IQ
- Findings
  - **Mild to profound mental retardation; learning problems**
  - **Large ears, dysmorphic facial features, large jaw, long face**
  - **Large testes—mostly in puberty (macroorchidism)(fertile)**
- Natural history—normal lifespan

EARLY OVERGROWTH WITH ASSOCIATED DEFECTS

Beckwith-Wiedemann Syndrome

- Genetics
  - Usually sporadic
  - IGF-2 disrupted at 11p15.5 (imprinted segment)
- Findings
  - **Macrosomia**
  - **Macroglossia—may need partial glossectomy**
  - **Pancreatic beta cell hyperplasia—excess islets → hypoglycemia;** hypoglycemia may be refractory; glucose control most important initial management
  - Umbilical abnormalities, diastasis recti, **omphalocele**
  - **Hemihypertrophy** → increased risk of abdominal tumors (Wilms)
- **Management—obtain ultrasounds and serum AFP every 6 months through 6 years of age to look for Wilms tumor and hepatoblastoma**

UNUSUAL BRAIN AND/OR NEUROMUSCULAR FINDINGS WITH ASSOCIATED DEFECTS

Prader-Willi Syndrome

- Genetics
  - Most with deletion at 15q11-q13–imprinted segment
  - **Paternal** chromosome responsible
  - The **same deletion** causes both Prader-Willi and Angelman syndromes. This may be due to the **normal process of imprinting**, which is **epigenetic** (change in the chromatin and not the gene sequence) silencing (due to hypermethylation) of certain genes in either the male or female germ cells. The alleles in the opposite

germ line are expressed and therefore in the zygote this results in **monoallelic gene expression** so that for any imprinted segment there is a **functional haploid state**. It is established in the germ line and maintained in all somatic cells.

- ○ If the deletion occurs in the **male germ cell**, then the inheritance is from the only expressed genes, which are maternal. This is Prader-Willi syndrome.
- ○ If the deletion occurs in the **female germ cell**, then the inheritance is from the only expressed genes, which are paternal. This is Angelman syndrome.

- – Negligible recurrence risk
- Findings
  - – First year, difficulty feeding with poor growth; then, increased feeding and weight gain plus slow height attainment (short stature)
  - – **Obesity—onset from 6 months to 6 years**
  - – **Mild to severe mental retardation**
  - – **Food-related behavioral problems (binge eating)**
  - – **Small hands and feet, puffy; small genitalia**
  - – **Hypothalamic—pituitary dysfunction (growth, thyroid, adrenal) hypogonadotrophic-hypogonadism**
- Natural history—decreased life expectancy relative to morbid obesity

Angelman Syndrome (Happy Puppet Syndrome)

- Genetics—also deletion of 15q11q13, but **maternally derived** (imprinted segment)
- Findings
  - – **Severe MR**
  - – **Paroxysms of inappropriate laughter**
  - – **Absent speech or <6 words (100%); most can communicate with sign language**
  - – **Ataxia and jerky arm movements resembling a puppet's movements (100%)**
  - – Seizures—most at age 4 years, may stop by age 10

FACIAL FEATURES AS THE MAJOR DEFECT

Robin Sequence (Pierre Robin)

- Mandibular hypoplasia in utero → posteriorly placed tongue → posterior palatal, shelves → cleft palate and other palatal abnormalities
- Isolated finding or associated with some syndromes/malformations—fetal alcohol syndrome, Edwards Syndrome
- Findings
  - – **Micrognathia**
  - – **Retroglossia → possible airway obstruction**
  - – **Cleft soft palate and other abnormalities**
- Jaw growth over first years of life if it results from a deformation; if part of a malformation syndrome, then it is a fixed finding

OSTEOCHONDRODYSPLASIAS

Achondroplasia/Hypochondroplasia

- Genetics
  - Autosomal dominant
  - Most common short-limb dwarfism
  - 90% from new gene mutation
  - Older paternal age
  - Mutations in gene for fibroblast growth factor receptor 3 at 4p16.3 (*FGFR3*)
- Findings
  - **Short stature (increased upper-to-lower segment ratio; short-limbed dwarfism)**
  - **Proximal femur shortening**
  - **Megalocephaly, small foramen magnum (may have hydrocephalus), small cranial base, prominent forehead**
  - **Lumbar lordosis**
- Natural history
  - Normal intelligence
  - Spinal cord compression is rare (cervicomedullary junction); usually occurs in first year of life
  - Tendency of late childhood obesity
  - Small eustachian tube—otitis media and hearing loss
  - Early cervical compression, respiratory problems, obstructive and central apnea, later cardiovascular disease

CONNECTIVE TISSUE DISORDERS

Marfan Syndrome

- Genetics
  - Autosomal dominant with wide variability
  - Mutation in fibrillin gene (*FBN1*)—15q21.1
- Findings
  - Early rapid growth of the appendicular skeleton and anterior ribs
  - Major findings are skeletal, cardiovascular, and ocular
  - **Tall stature with long, slim limbs and little fat**
  - Arm span > height
  - **Arachnodactyly** long slender fingers and toes
  - Decreased U:L segment ratio (as with XXY) U:L = upper to lower body
  - **Joint laxity with kyphoscoliosis**
  - Pectus excavatum or carinatum
  - **Lens subluxation (upward; defect in suspensory ligament)**; secondary glaucoma, myopia, retinal detachment

- **Ascending aortic dilatation with or without dissecting aneurysm** (uncommon in children and adolescents unless case is severe) with secondary aortic regurgitation. Mitral valve disease (MVP and regurgitation) is the most common in children.
- Natural history
  - Prevent scoliosis
  - Vascular complications chief cause of death
  - Evaluate heart and aorta

Ehlers-Danlos Syndrome

- Genetics
  - Type I most common (now 6 types)
  - Autosomal dominant with wide variability
- Findings
  - **Droopy ears**
  - **Hyperextensible skin, fragile, easy bruisability, poor wound healing**
  - **Joint hyperlaxity; tendency toward hip, shoulder, knee, and clavicular dislocation**
  - MVP, tricuspid valve prolapse, **aortic root dilatation;** dissecting aneurysm, ASD
  - **Blue sclera**, myopia, glaucoma, **ectopia lentis**, retinal detachment
  - Intracranial aneurysm

ENVIRONMENTAL AGENTS

Fetal Alcohol Syndrome (FAS)

- Alcohol—most common teratogen to which fetus can be exposed
- Findings—variable
  - **Pre- (symmetric IUGR) and postnatal growth deficiency (short stature)**
  - **Mental retardation, microcephaly**
  - Fine motor dysfunction
  - Irritability in infancy, **hyperactivity in childhood**
  - **Behavioral abnormalities**
  - **Mid-face dysmorphism (abnormal frontal lobe development)**, short palpebral fissures, maxillary hypoplasia, short nose, smooth philtrum, thin and smooth upper lip
  - **Joint abnormalities**—abnormal position and/or function
  - **Cardiac anomalies: VSD > ASD**, tetralogy of Fallot

Fetal Hydantoin Syndrome

- **Similar features with prenatal exposure to carbamazepine, valproate, primidone, and phenobarbital**
- **No dose-response relationship has been demonstrated**
- Growth deficiency

Note

Etiology of FAS
Severity of maternal alcohol use and extent and severity of pattern is most predictive of ultimate prognosis.

- Borderline to mild mental retardation
- Dysmorphic facial features; short neck; abnormal palmar crease
- Rib abnormalities
- **Hirsutism**
- **Cupid's-bow lips**

Fetal Valproate Syndrome

- **Midface hypoplasia;** cleft lip
- **Cardiac defects**
- Long, thin fingers and toes; convex nails
- **Meningomyelocele**

Retinoic Acid Embryopathy (from Isotretinoin)

- Mild facial asymmetry; **bilateral microtia/anotia (ear); facial nerve paralysis ipsilateral to ear;** narrow, sloping forehead; abnormal mottling of teeth
- **Conotruncal malformations**
- **CNS malformations**
- **Decreased intelligence**
- Thymic and parathyroid abnormalities
- **No problems if stopped before 15th postmenstrual day**
- Pregnancy test required prior to treatment with isotretinoin

MISCELLANEOUS SEQUENCES

Potter Sequence

- Etiology
  - **Renal agenesis/dysgenesis** or other type of urinary tract defect must occur prior to 31 days' gestation → **oligohydramnios** (also from chronic leakage)
  - Leads to **fetal compression (mid-face, ears)**
  - Lack of alveolar sac development → **pulmonary hypoplasia**
- Findings
  - **Pulmonary hypoplasia**
  - **Potter facies**—hypertelorism, epicanthal folds, low-set flattened ears, micrognathia, compressed flat nose
  - Breech presentation
  - Abnormal positioning of hands and feet; deformations, limb anomalies
  - **Death from respiratory insufficiency (hypoplasia)**

Note

All females who are to be treated with isotretinoin must:

- Take pregnancy test
- Use definitive method of birth control (e.g., OCPs)
- Use one back-up method of birth control (e.g., condoms)
- Receive counseling regarding teratogenicity

Note

An U/S is necessary for the parents and siblings of patients with oligohydramnios secondary to agenesis and/or dysgenesis of both kidneys. This is because 9% of first-degree relatives have asymptomatic malformations.

MISCELLANEOUS ASSOCIATIONS

VACTERL Association

- Nonrandom association of
    - V = Vertebral defects
    - A = Anal atresia (imperforate anus)
    - C = Cardiac defects (VSD and others)
    - T = TE fistula
    - E = Esophageal atresia
    - R = Renal defects
    - L = Limb defects (radial)

CHARGE Association

- Nonrandom association of
    - C = Coloboma (from isolated iris to anophthalmos; retinal most common)
    - H = Heart defects (TOF, PDA, and others)
    - A = Atresia choanae
    - R = Retardation of growth and/or development
    - G = Genital hypoplasia (in males)
    - E = Ear anomalies and/or deafness

Growth and Nutrition 3

Learning Objectives

❏ Demonstrate steps in evaluation of growth

❏ Solve problems related to breast feeding, feeding of solids, and other feeding issues

❏ Answer questions related to growth disorders

CHILDHOOD GROWTH

Basic Principles of Growth

- A newborn typically loses **up to 10% of birth weight (BW) in the first week of life** due to elimination of large amount of extravascular fluid. **Should regain or surpass BW by 2 weeks.**

- A neonate should gain about 30 grams (1 oz) per day in the first month of life, which slows to about 20 grams/day at 3–4 months.

- **An infant typically doubles BW by 6 months and triples by 1 year.**

- Growth rate slows further between 6 and 12 months and then appetite begins to decline through 18 months of age.

- Then height and weight increase at a steady rate, but head-circumference rate of growth decreases somewhat (2–5 years).

- Between age 6 and 12 years: **3–6 growth spurts** each year for 8 week periods each; slower brain growth; **myelination complete by age 7**

- Between age 10 and 20 years: acceleration in early adolescence. Boys' highest growth stops at age 18. **Their average peak is 13.5 years (2–3 years later than girls, and continues 2–3 years after girls have stopped).** Girls' **average peak is 11.5 years and it stops at age 16.**

Assessment of Growth

- Child is genetically programmed to stay on 1–2 growth curves after age 2 years.

- Height percentile at age 2 years correlates with final adult height percentile.

- Low-birth-weight and very-low-birth-weight infants may continue to show **catch-up growth through early school age.**

- **Weight/height <5th percentile is the single best growth curve indicator for acute malnutrition.** In nutritional insufficiency, weight decreases before length, and weight/height is low. For causes of decreased linear growth, length decreases first or at the same time as weight (e.g., GH deficiency).

- **BMI is accepted as best clinical indicator for measure of under- and overweight.**
- For bone age-reference standards, use **radiographs of left hand and wrist. Skeletal maturity is linked more to sexual maturity than chronologic age.**

Growth Patterns

The **growth chart is the best tool to determine patterns of growth.** There are separate growth charts for boys and girls. The **charts measure weight for age, height for age, head circumference for age, weight for height, and body mass index (BMI).**

- Each chart has multiple curves (either 5–95% or 3–97%).

Evaluation of Growth

Definitions

- **Growth velocity (GV)**—yearly increments of growth; should follow a growth curve

$$\text{slope} = \frac{\text{change in height}}{\text{change in age}}$$

- **Chronologic age (CA)**—actual age
- **Bone age (BA)**—x-ray of left hand and wrist (non-dominant hand)

Table 3-1. Growth Velocity

	Normal	Abnormal
Bone age = Chronological age,	Ideal Genetic (familial) **short stature**	• Genetic • Chromosomal
Bone age < Chronological age	Constitutional delay	• Chronic systemic disease • Endocrine related
Bone age ≥ Chronological age	Obesity (tall) Familial **tall stature**	• Precocious puberty • Congenital adrenal hyperplasia • Hyperthyroidism

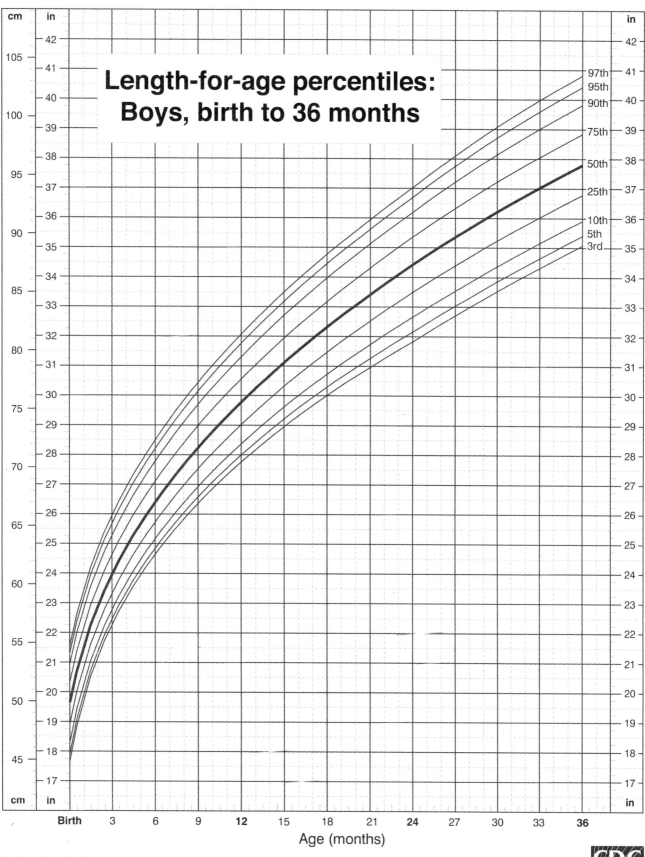

Length-for-age percentiles: Boys, birth to 36 months

Age (months)

Published May 30, 2000.
SOURCE: Developed by the National Center for Health Statistics in collaboration with
the National Center for Chronic Disease Prevention and Health Promotion (2000).

CDC
SAFER · HEALTHIER · PEOPLE™

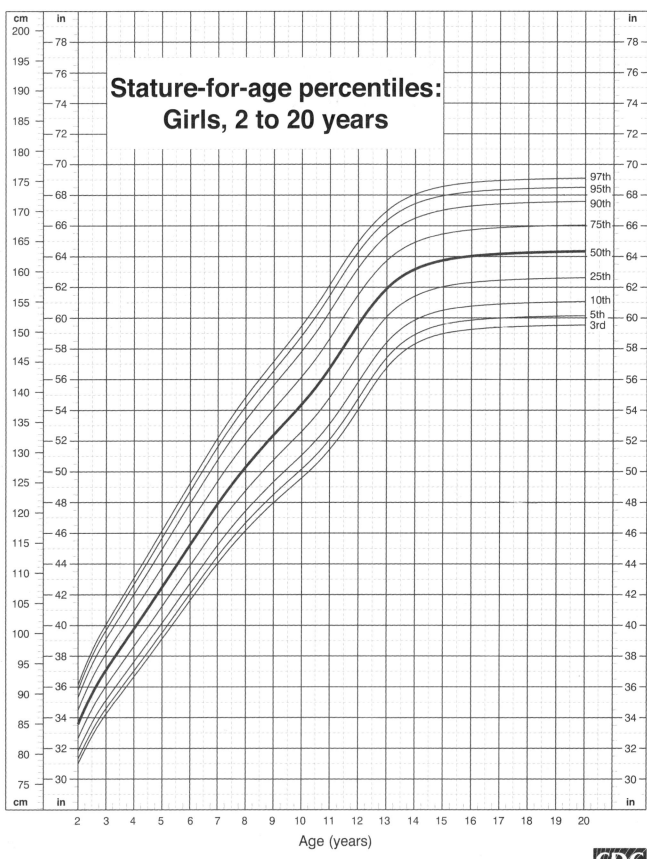

Stature-for-age percentiles: Girls, 2 to 20 years

Age (years)

Published May 30, 2000.
SOURCE: Developed by the National Center for Health Statistics in collaboration with
the National Center for Chronic Disease Prevention and Health Promotion (2000).

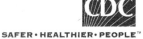

SAFER ● HEALTHIER ● PEOPLE™

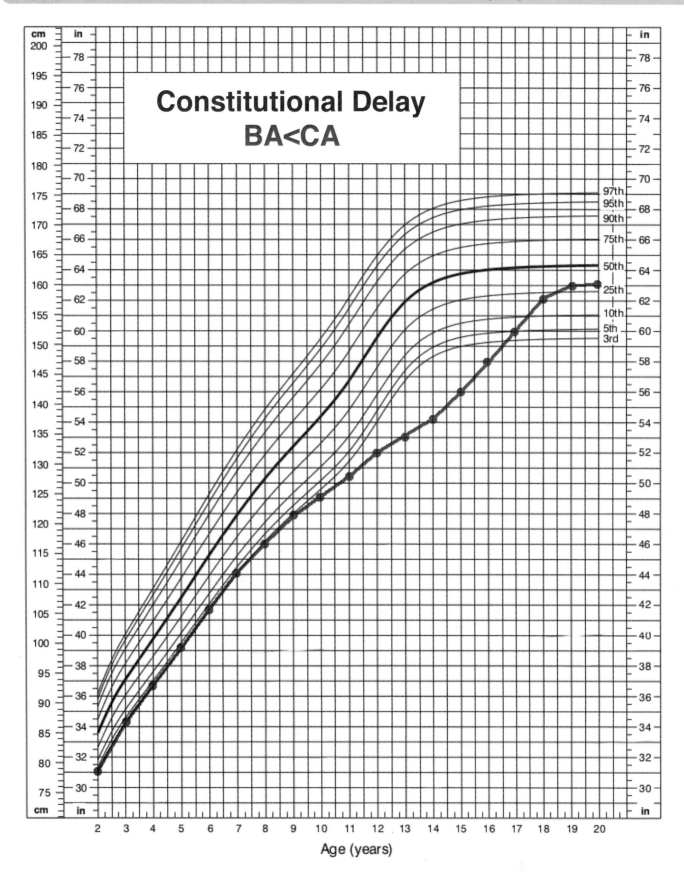

Constitutional Delay
BA<CA

Adapted from CDC.gov/National Center for Health Statistics

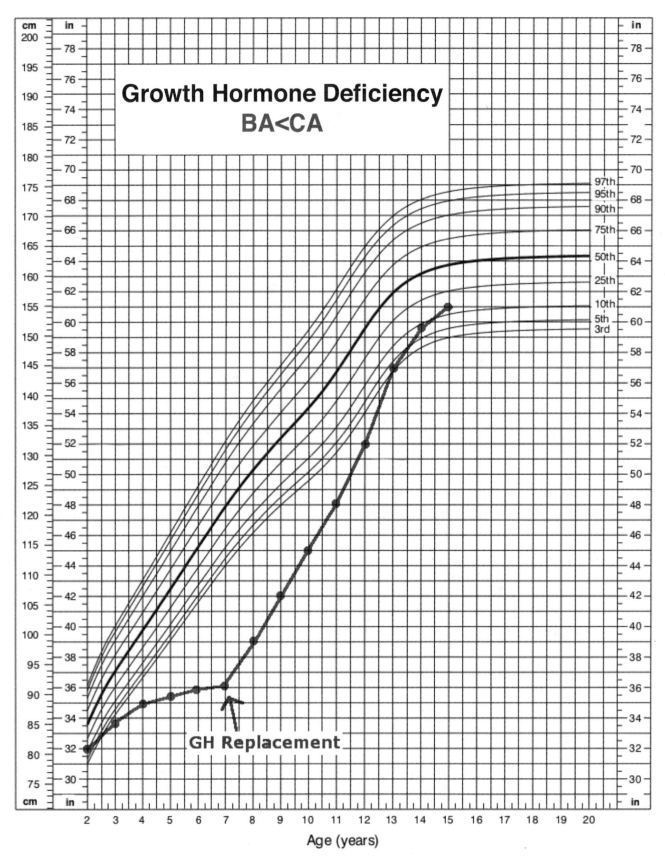

Growth Hormone Deficiency
BA<CA

GH Replacement

Adapted from CDC.gov/National Center for Health Statistics

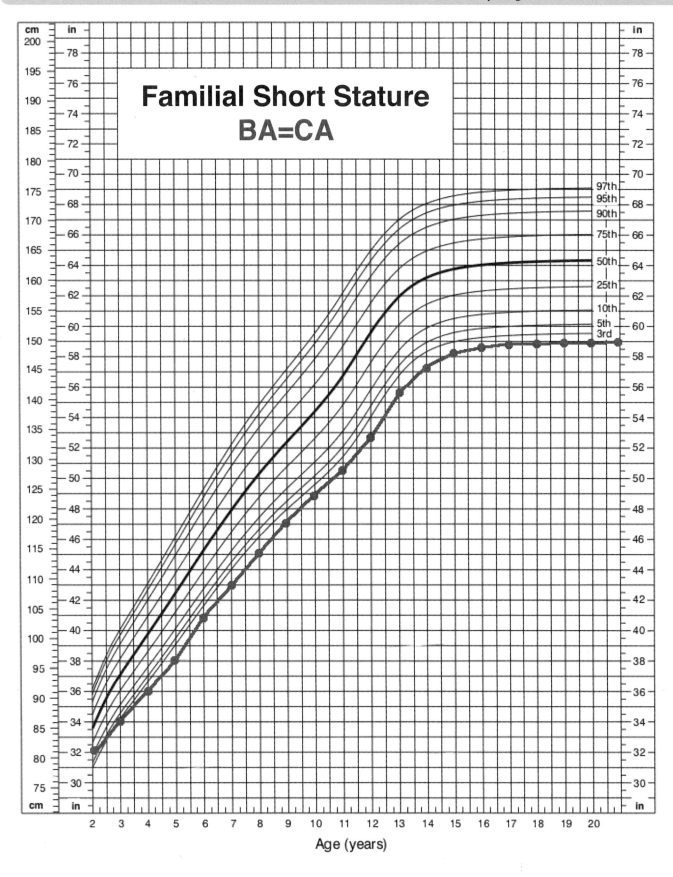

Familial Short Stature
BA=CA

Age (years)

Adapted from CDC.gov/National Center for Health Statistics

DISORDERS OF GROWTH

Height

Note

Suspect *Turner syndrome* in females with pathologic short stature.

Suspect *craniopharyngioma* if short stature and vision problems.

Short stature

A father is worried that his 13-year-old son is short. The child has been very healthy. He is below the fifth percentile for height and has been all his life. Physical exam is normal. Father is 6 foot 3; mother is 5 foot 10. Father was a "late bloomer."

- Constitutional growth delay—child is short prior to onset of delayed adolescent growth spurt; parents are of normal height; normal final adult height is reached; growth spurt and puberty are delayed; bone age delayed compared to chronological age.
- Familial short stature—patient is parallel to growth curve; strong family history of short stature; chronologic age equals bone age.
- Pathologic short stature—patient may start out in normal range but then starts crossing growth percentiles. Differential diagnosis: craniopharyngioma, hypothyroidism, hypopituitarism, nutritional problems, and other chronic illnesses.

Tall stature

- Usually a normal variant (familial tall stature)
- Other causes—exogenous obesity, endocrine causes (growth hormone excess [gigantism, acromegaly], androgen excess [tall as children, short as adults)
- Syndromes—homocystinuria, Sotos, Klinefelter

Weight

Organic failure to thrive

A baby weighs 16 pounds at 1 year of age. Birth weight was 8 pounds. Parents state that the baby feeds well. Physical exam reveals a baby with little subcutaneous fat, long dirty fingernails, impetigo, and a flat occiput.

- Malnutrition
  - Malabsorption (infection, celiac disease, cystic fibrosis, disaccharide deficiency, protein-losing enteropathy)
  - Allergies
  - Immunodeficiency
  - Chronic disease
- Initial diagnostic tests (when organic causes are suspected)—**document caloric intake,** CBC, urinalysis, liver function tests, serum protein, **sweat chloride**, stool for ova and parasites

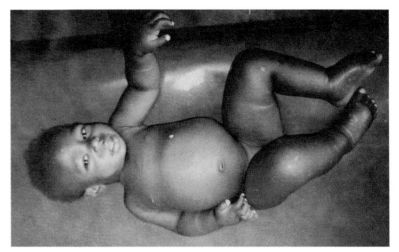

Courtesy of Tom D. Thacher, M.D.

Figure 3-1. Kwashiorkor
Note generalized edema secondary to low serum albumin.

Non-organic failure to thrive

A 4-month-old infant presents to the emergency department because of upper respiratory symptoms. The patient is <5 percentile in weight and length. He is 3.5 kg. Birth weight was 4.2 kg. The mother states that the patient takes 16 oz of infant formula per day with cereal added.

- Child (usually infant) not fed adequate calories
  - Emotional or maternal deprivation concurrent with nutritional deprivation
  - Leads to neglect of infant; psychosocial deprivation most common reason in all age groups
  - Other factors: retarded or emotionally disturbed parents; poverty
- Clinical findings
  - Thin extremities, narrow face, prominent ribs, wasted buttocks
  - Neglect of hygiene
  - A flat occiput and hair loss may indicate excessive back-lying
  - Delays in social and speech development
  - Avoidance of eye contact, expressionless, no cuddling response
  - Feeding aversions
- Diagnosis—Feed under supervision (may need hospitalization) for 1 week.
  - Should gain >2 oz/24 hours over the week
  - May have a ravenous appetite
  - Careful observations of mother; may need videotape
  - Delay extensive lab evaluations until after dietary management has been attempted for 1 week and has failed.

- Management
  - **All cases caused by underfeeding from maternal neglect must be reported to CPS**
  - **Infants discharged to natural home require intensive and long-term intervention**
  - Feed, as above; usually require greater calories for catch-up growth. May need NG feedings or even gastrostomy tube in severe cases

Obesity

- Risk factors—predisposition, parental obesity, family/patient inactivity, feeding baby as response to any crying, and rarely associated in syndromes (Prader-Willi; Down)
- Presentation—tall stature in some, abdominal striae, associated obesity of extremities; increased adipose tissue in mammary tissue in boys, large pubic fat pad, early puberty
- Diagnostic tests
  - BMI >95% for age and sex is diagnostic of obesity
  - 85 to 95% = overweight
- Complications—Obese infants and children are at increased risk of becoming obese adults (the risk is greater with advanced age of onset); cardiovascular (hypertension, increased cholesterol), hyperinsulinism, slipped capital femoral epithesis, sleep apnea, type 2 diabetes, acanthosis nigrans.
- Treatment—exercise and balanced diet; **no medications**

FEEDING

- **Normal newborn has sufficient stores of iron to meet requirements for 4–6 months,** but iron stores and absorption are variable. **Breast milk has less iron than most formulas, but has higher bioavailability.**
- **Formula is supplemented with vitamin D; breast fed must be supplemental from birth (400 IU/d).**
- **Vitamin K routinely is given IM (intramuscularly) at birth**, so supplementation is not needed.
- Breast milk and formula are 90% H20, so no additional H2O needed

BREAST FEEDING

A nursing mother asks if her 3-month-old baby requires any vitamin supplementation.

- Most infants can breast feed immediately after birth and all can feed by 4–6 months. The feeding schedule should be by self-regulation; most establish by 1 month.
- Advantages
  - Psychological/emotional—maternal-infant bonding
  - Premixed; right temperature and concentration
  - Immunity—**protective effects** against enteric and other pathogens; **less diarrhea, intestinal bleeding, spitting up, early unexplained infant crying, atopic dermatitis, allergy, and chronic illnesses** later in life; passive transfer of T-cell immunity
  - Decreased allergies compared to formula fed
  - Maternal—weight loss and faster return to preconceptional uterine size

Note

Mothers with HBV infection are free to breast feed their infants **after** the neonate has received the appropriate recommended vaccinations against HBV.

- Contraindications
  - HIV
  - CMV, HSV (if lesions on breast)
  - HBV (*see* note)
  - Acute maternal disease if infant does not have disease (tuberculosis, sepsis)
  - Breast cancer
  - Substance abuse
  - Drugs: (**absolute contraindications**) antineoplastics, radiopharmaceuticals, ergot alkaloids, iodide/mercurials, atropine, lithium, chloramphenicol, cyclosporin, nicotine, alcohol; (**relative contraindications**) neuroleptics, sedatives, tranquilizers, metronidazole, tetracycline, sulfonamides, steroids
  - Breast feeding is *not* contraindicated in mastitis.

Table 3-2. Comparison of Breast Milk to Cow Milk

Component	Human Milk	Cow Milk
Water/solids	Same	Same
Calories	20 cal/oz	20 cal/oz
Protein	1–1.5% (whey dominant)	3.3% (casein dominant)
Carbohydrate	6.5–7% lactose	4.5% lactose
Fat	high in low chain fatty acids	high in medium chain fatty acids
Minerals	Iron better absorbed	Low iron and copper
Vitamins	Diet dependent, low in K	Low in C, D
Digestibility	Faster emptying	Same after 45 days
Renal solute load	**Low** (aids in renal function)	Higher

Formula Feeding

- **Infant formulas.** Formula feeding is used to **substitute** or **supplement** breast milk. Most commercial formulas are cow-milk–based with modifications to approximate breast milk. They contain **20 calories/ounce.** Specialty formulas (soy, lactose-free, premature, elemental) are modified to meet specific needs.
- Formula versus cow milk—**Fe-deficiency anemia with early introduction (<1 yr) of cow's milk**
- Advanced feeding—Stepwise addition of foods (one new food every 3–4 days)

Note

Do not give cow milk to infants age <1.

SOLIDS

- Iron-fortified cereal only at 4-6 months
- Step-wise introduction of strained foods (vegetables and fruits), then dairy, meats (6-9 months; stage I and II)
- Table foods at 9-12 months
  - Foods better saved for year 2:
    - Egg whites
    - Nuts
    - Wheat products
    - Chocolate
    - Citrus
    - Fish
  - No honey in first year of life—infant botulism

Development 4

Learning Objectives

❑ Explain information related to primitive reflexes and developmental milestones

OVERVIEW

- Five main skill areas
  - Visual-motor
  - Language
  - Motor
  - Social
  - Adaptive
- Assessment based on acquisition of milestones occurring sequentially and at a specific rate
  - Each skill area has a spectrum of normal and abnormal.
  - Abnormal development in one area increases likelihood of abnormality in another—**so need to do a careful assessment of all skills**
  - Developmental diagnosis—functional description/classification; does *not* specify an etiology
- Developmental delay—performance significantly below average, i.e., developmental quotient (developmental age/chronologic age × 100) of <75
  - May be in one or more areas
  - Two assessments over time are more predictive than a single assessment
- Major developmental disorders
  - Mental retardation—**IQ <70–75 *plus* related limitation in at least 2 adaptive skills**, e.g., self-care, home living, work, communication
  - Communication disorders (deficits of comprehension, interpretation, production, or use of language)
  - Learning disabilities, one or more of (defined by federal government; based on standardized tests): reading, listening, speaking, writing, math
  - Cerebral palsy
  - Attention deficit/hyperactivity disorder
  - Autism spectrum disorders

Medical Evaluation

- Thorough history and physical
- Developmental testing—age-appropriate motor, visual, cognitive, language, behavioral and learning
- Denver II Developmental Assessment
  - Tool for screening the apparently normal child between ages 0–6
  - Suggested at every well-child care visit
  - Allows generalist to identify possible delay → need further evaluation for definitive diagnosis
  - Screens in gross motor, fine motor, language, personal-social
  - **For infants born <38 weeks' gestation, correct age for prematurity up to age 2 years**
  - Failure is at least 2 delays

PRIMITIVE REFLEXES AND DEVELOPMENTAL MILESTONES

An infant can sit up with its back straight, has started crawling, has a pincer grasp, and plays peek-a-boo. What age is most appropriate for this baby?

- Appear and disappear in sequence during specific periods of development
- **Absence or persistence beyond a given time frame signifies CNS dysfunction**

Included here are the major milestones indicative of specific ages. Exam questions typically describe an infant's/child's skills and ask for the corresponding age.

Table 4-1. Newborn Reflexes

Reflex	Description	Appears	Disappears	CNS Origin
Moro	Extend head → extension, flexion of arms, legs	Birth	4–6 mo	Brain stem vestibular nuclei
Grasp	Finger in palm → hand, elbow, shoulder flexion	Birth	4–6 mo	Brain stem vestibular nuclei
Rooting	Cheek stimulus → turns mouth to that side	Birth	4–6 mo	Brain stem trigeminal system
Trunk incurvation	Withdrawal from stroking along ventral surface	Birth	6–9 mo	Spinal cord
Placing	Steps up when dorsum of foot stimulated	Birth	4–6 mo	Cerebral cortex
Asymmetric tonic neck (ATNR)	Fencing posture when supine	Birth to 1 month	4–6 mo	Brain stem vestibular nuclei
Parachute	Simulate fall → extends arms	6–8 mo	Never	Brain stem vestibular

Table 4-2. Developmental Milestones

	Gross Motor	Visual Motor	Language	Social Adaptive
Birth	• Symmetric movements in supine • Head flat in prone	• Visually fixes on an object	• Alerts to sound	• Regards face
2 months	• Head in midline while held sitting • Raises head in prone • Begins to lift chest	• Follows past midline	• Smiles in response to touch and voice	• Recognizes parent
4 months	• Holds head steadily • Supports on forearms in prone • Rolls from prone to supine	• Reaches with both arms together • Hands to midline	• Laughs • Orients to voice • Coos	• Likes to look around
6 months	• Sits with support (tripod) • Feet in mouth in supine	• Unilateral reach • Raking grasp • Transfers object	• Babbles	• Recognizes that someone is a stranger
7 months	• Rolls from supine to prone • May crawl • Starts to sit without support			
9 months	• Crawls well • Pulls to stand • Starting to cruise	• Immature pincer grasp • Holds bottle • Throws object (not overhand)	• "Mama," "dada," indiscriminately • Understands "no" • Understands gestures	• Plays gesture games • Explores environment (crawling and cruising)
12 months	• May walk alone (must by 18 months)	• Mature pincer grasp • Crayon marks • Object permanence (from 10 months)	• 1-2 words other than "mama" and "dada" (used appropriately) • Follows 1-step command with gesture	• Imitates actions • Comes when called • Cooperates with dressing
15 months	• Creeps up stairs • Walks backward	• Scribbles and builds towers of 2 blocks in imitation	• 4-6 words • Follows 1-step command without gesture	• Uses cup and spoon (variable until 18 months)
18 months	• Runs • Throws objects overhand while standing	• Scribbles spontaneously • Builds tower of 3 blocks	• 15-25 words • Knows 5 body parts	• Imitates parents in tasks • Plays in company of other children

(Continued)

Table 4-2. Developmental Milestones (*Cont'd*)

	Gross Motor	Visual Motor	Language	Social Adaptive
24 months	• Walks up, and down stairs one foot at a time	• Imitates stroke (up or down) with pencil • Builds tower of 7 blocks • Removes clothing	• 50 words • 2-word sentences • Follows 2-step commands • Uses pronouns inappropriately	• Parallel play
3 years	• Alternates feet going up the stairs • Pedals tricycle	• Copies a circle • Undresses completely • Dresses partially • Unbuttons • Dries hands	• ≥250 words • 3-word sentences • Plurals • All pronouns	• Group play • Shares • Takes turns • Knows full name, age and gender
4 years	• Alternates feet going downstairs • Hops and skips	• Copies a square • Buttons clothing • Dresses completely • Catches ball	• Knows colors • Recites songs from memory • Asks questions	• Plays cooperatively • Tells "tall tales"
5 years	• Skips alternating feet • Jumps over lower obstacles	• Copies triangle • Ties shoes • Spreads with knife	• Prints first name • Asks what a word means • Answers all "wh-" questions • Tells a story • Plays pretend • Knows alphabet	• Plays cooperative games • Abides by rules • Likes to help in household tasks

Possible Abnormalities

You must take into account the number of weeks of prematurity to assess development appropriately, i.e., per the preterm age, NOT chronological. For instance, a 6-month-old baby born at 32 weeks (i.e., 2 months preterm) must be assessed at 6 − 2 = 4 months CORRECTED AGE. Do this until chronological age 2 years, then consider delays to be true.

- If there appears to be a language delay, first consider conductive hearing loss. While all babies receive hearing testing within the first month of life, that is for congenital sensorineural hearing loss. Over the first year of life, conductive hearing loss may occur from repeated ear infections.

- If there is a lack of development or regression of language skills with impaired social interaction, restricted activities and interests and stereotypic behaviors, consider autistic spectrum disorder. Onset of abnormal findings must occur age <3 years.

  - After a complete H and P with neurologic exam and development testing, the first step is to perform an autism screening questionnaire. If you feel the diagnosis is likely, the next step is to refer to a specialist in this area.

- Delay is defined as ≥1 **skills significantly below average**, i.e., developmental quotient (developmental age/chronological age x 100) is <75. When you find this, you must first look for a possible reason, and the child will need developmental therapy in ≥1 areas.

Behavioral/Psychological Disorders 5

Learning Objectives

❏ Solve problems concerning eating disorders, elimination disorders, and sleep disorders

EATING DISORDERS

Pica

- Repeated or chronic ingestion of non-nutritive substances, e.g., paint, dirt
- After year 2, needs investigation
- Predisposing factors
  - **Mental retardation and lack of parental nurturing**
  - Also with family disorganization, poor supervision, and psychologic neglect
- More common with autism, brain-behavior disorders, and **low socioeconomic status**
- Increased risk for **lead poisoning, iron deficiency, and parasitic infections**

ELIMINATION DISORDERS

Enuresis

A 7-year old boy has problems with bedwetting. The mother says that during the day he has no problems but is usually wet 6 of 7 mornings. He does not report dysuria or frequency, and has not had increased thirst. The mother also says that he is a deep sleeper.

- Definition—voluntary or involuntary repeated discharge of urine after a developmental age when bladder control should be present (most by age of **5 years**); there are 2 types
- **Primary:**
  - **No significant dry period**; most common and usually **nocturnal** (nocturnal enuresis)
  - Hyposecretion of ADH and/or receptor dysfunction

- Relationship of sleep architecture, diminished arousability during sleep, and abnormal bladder function; anatomic malformations
- Management—thorough history and physical, (should begin with behavioral treatment; not definitive, varying success rates):
  ○ Enlist cooperation of child—chart dryness, reward system
  ○ Child should void before going to sleep
  ○ Alarm to wake once 2–3 hours after falling asleep; may use alarm that goes off when child wets a special sheet (bell and pad alarm)
  ○ No punishment or humiliation
  ○ Psychotherapy for traumatized children or when behavioral therapy has failed
  ○ Pharmacotherapy for failed behavioral therapy in nocturnal enuresis— oral desmopressin (DDAVP)
- **Secondary**:
  - **After a period of dryness ≥6 months**
  - Causes—psychological, urinary tract infection, constipation, diabetes
  - More common in girls
  - Evaulation—urinalysis
  - Management—treat underlying disorder
- **Children with both diurnal and nocturnal enuresis:**
  - Especially with voiding difficulties, more likely to have abnormalities of the urinary tract
  - Ultrasonography or flow studies are indicated in these cases.

Encopresis

- Definition—passage of feces into inappropriate places after a chronologic age of 4 years, or equivalent developmental level
- May be primary or secondary
- Causes—psychological (toilet phobia), early toilet training, agressive management of constipation, painful defecation, fissures
- Types
  - Retentive encopresis most common:
    ○ 2/3 of cases
    ○ **Hard stool on rectal examination is sufficient to document**, but a negative exam requires a plain abdominal x-ray
    ○ Presence of fecal retention is evidence of chronic constipation, and thus treatment will require **active constipation management**
    ○ May have abnormal anal sphincter function
- Associations
  - Primary encopresis—especially in boys, associated with global developmental delays and enuresis
  - Secondary encopresis—high levels of psychosocial stressors and conduct disorder

- Management
  - **First—clear impacted fecal material and short-term use of mineral oil or laxatives. No long-term laxative use**
  - Concomitant behavioral management
  - Regular postprandial toilet-sitting
  - High-fiber diet
  - Familial support for behavior modification
  - Group or individual psychotherapy

SLEEP DISORDERS

Parasomnias

- Definition—**episodic** nocturnal behaviors that often involve cognitive disorientation and autonomic and skeletal muscle disturbance
- Associated with relative CNS immaturity
- More common in children than adults; abates with age

Table 5-1. Parasomnias

Sleepwalking and Sleep Terrors (Partial Arousal)	Nightmares
• First third of night	• Last third of night
• During slow-wave sleep	• REM sleep
• **No daytime sleepiness or recall**	• **Daytime sleepiness** (if prolonged waking) and **vivid recall**
• High arousal threshold (agitated if • awakened)	• **Low arousal threshold** (easily awakened)
• **Common family history**	• No family history
• Displaced from bed	• May be displaced from bed
• Sleepwalking relatively common; night terrors rare	• Very common
• Treatment: parental education, **reassurance**, avoid exacerbating factors, i.e., sleep deprivation, **safety precautions**	• No required treatment unless persistent/frequent, in which case possible abuse or anxiety disorder should be investigated.

Learning Objectives

❑ Define active immunization

❑ Describe different routes of immunization for specific routine vaccines

A 6-month-old patient is being seen for routine care. The baby is doing well, and physical examination, growth, and development are normal. The mother states that after the last set of immunizations the baby had a temperature of 39.4°C (103°F) and cried for 2 hours but was consolable. What is your advice to this mother before administering the next set of immunizations?

ACTIVE IMMUNIZATIONS

Table 6-1. Classification of Vaccines

Live Attenuated		
	• Viral	MMR, varicella, yellow fever, nasal influenza, smallpox, oral rotavirus
	• Bacterial	BCG, oral typhoid
Inactivated		
Whole	• Virus	Polio, rabies, hepatitis A
Fractional	• Protein-based	Subunit: hepatitis B, parenteral influenza, acellular pertussis
	• Polysaccharide based	Toxoid: diphtheria, tetanus
		Pure: pneumococcal, Hib, meningococcal
		Conjugate: Hib, pneumococcal, meningococcal

Vaccine Rules

- For stimulation of an adequate and persisting antibody response, 2 or more doses are usually required.
- Interchangeability of vaccine products—in general, most vaccines from different manufacturers may be interchangeable.

- Simultaneous administration—most can be safely and effectively given simultaneously.
- Lapsed immunizations—**a lapse in schedule does not require reinstitution of the entire series**.
- Unknown or uncertain immunization status
    - **When in doubt, the child should be considered to be disease-susceptible, and appropriate immunizations should be initiated without delay.**
    - **To be counted, the vaccine(s) must be documented on a formal immunization record, regardless of country.**
- Dose—No reduced dose or divided dose should be administered, **including to babies born prematurely or at low birth weight (exception: first dose hepatitis B).**
- Active immunization of people who recently received gamma globulin
    - **Live virus vaccine may have diminished immunogenicity when given shortly before or during the several months after receipt of immunoglobulin (Ig) so live vaccine is delayed (3–11 months).**

Institute of Medicine Immunization Safety Review Committee findings

- Available evidence **does not support the hypothesis that the MMR causes autism, associated disorders, or inflammatory bowel disease**. (Lancet report of Wakefield has been found to be fraudulent)
- Based on epidemiologic evidence, there is **no causal relationship between multiple immunizations and increased risk of immune dysfunction and type 1 diabetes.**
- There is no causal relationship between hepatitis B vaccine administration and demyelinating neurologic disorders.
- There is no causal relationship between meningococcal vaccination and Guillain-Barré.
- Preservative thimerosal (Hg-containing) not causative of any problems (has now been removed)

Misconceptions

The following are *not* contraindications to immunizations:

- A reaction to a previous DTaP of temperature <105°F, redness, soreness, and swelling
- A mild, acute illness in an otherwise well child
- Concurrent antimicrobial therapy
- Prematurity—immunize at the chronological age
- A family history of seizures
- A family history of sudden infant death syndrome

Accepted Precautions and Contraindications

- Minor illness, with or without a fever, **does not contraindicate immunization.**
- **Fever, per se, is not a contraindication.**
    - Guidelines for administration are based on the physician's assessment of illness and on specific vaccines the child is scheduled to receive.

- If fever or other problems suggest moderate or serious illness, the child should not be immunized until recovered.
- **Documented egg allergy is *not* a contraindication to the MMR.** MMR is derived from chick embryo fibroblast tissue cultures but *does not* contain significant amounts of egg cross-reacting proteins.
- **Influenza vaccine (and yellow fever) *does* contain egg protein** and on *rare* occasions may induce a significant immediate hypersensitivity reaction.

ACTIVE IMMUNIZATION AFTER DISEASE EXPOSURE

Measles

Table 6-2. Measles

Age	Management (post-exposure)
0–6 months	Immune serum globulin if mother is not immune
Pregnant or immunocompromised	Immune serum globulin
All others	Vaccine within 72 hours of exposure for susceptible individuals

Varicella

- Give vaccine **to susceptible immunocompetent contacts age >12 months as soon as possible and VZIG to all immunocompromised and susceptible pregnant women.** No vaccine or VZIG for healthy infants age 0-12 months.
- **VZIG also for** susceptible pregnant women, **newborn whose mother had the onset of chicken pox within 5 days before delivery to 48 hours after delivery,** and certain hospitalized premature infants

Hepatitis

- Hepatitis B: after exposure in nonimmune patient, give hepatitis B Ig plus vaccine; repeat vaccine at 1 and 6 months.
- Hepatitis A: if patient is not vaccinated, give 1 dose of vaccine as soon as possible but within 2 weeks of exposure

Mumps and Rubella

- Not protected by postexposure administration of live vaccine
- Recommended for exposed adults who were born in the United States in or since 1957 and who have not previously had or been immunized against either; except pregnancy

SPECIFIC VACCINES (ROUTINE VACCINATION)

Hepatitis B

- First dose should be given soon after birth, before hospital discharge, with a total of **3 doses by age 18 months** if mother is HBsAg negative.

- **The infant born to a hepititis B surface antigen (HBsAg)-positive mother should receive the first dose of hepatitis B virus (HBV) plus hepatitis B Ig at 2 different sites within 12 hours of birth;** all 3 doses should be given by age 6 months (treat same as exposure).

- All children and adolescents who have not been immunized should begin the series during any visit to the physician.

DTaP

- All DTaP vaccines for United States currently contain acellular **pertussis.**

- The rates of local reactions, fever, and other common systemic reactions are **substantially lower with acellular pertussis vaccines than with whole-cell vaccine (but may still occur).** Use DT if there has been a serious reaction and also for any catch-up after age 7 (i.e., no full dose pertussis after age 7).

- Total of 5 doses is recommended before school entry, with the final given at **preschool age, 4–6 years.**

- Pertussis booster (Tdap) vaccine **is now recommended during adolescence, regardless of immunization status; is also recommended even if one has already had pertussis disease.**

- Tdap (childhood tetanus) is given at **age 11–12**, and then Td (adult tetanus) every 10 years.

Tetanus

Table 6-3. Tetanus Prophylaxis in Wound Management

History of Doses of Tetanus Toxoid	Clean, Minor Wounds		All Others*	
	Td	**TIG**	**Td**	**TIG**
<3 or unknown	Yes	No	Yes	Yes
≥3	No, unless >10 years from last dose	No	No, unless >5 years from last dose	No

Definition of abbreviations: TIG, tetanus immune globulin; Td, tetanus and diptheria vaccine.

*All other wounds = increased risk of tetanus: dirt, saliva, feces, avulsions, frostbite, puncture, crush, burns, and missiles.

IPV

- Inactivated is now the **only poliovirus vaccine available in the United States**.

- Four doses of IPV, with the last at **preschool age, 4–6 years**

- Any child up to 18 years of age should receive all doses, if behind.

- Any child who has received OPV from another country should complete schedule in United States with IPV.

HiB Conjugated Vaccine

- *Does not* cover nontypeable *Haemophilus*
- Depending on the vaccine brand, the recommended primary series consists of 3 or 4 doses.
- After the primary series, an additional booster dose is recommended at 12–15 months of age, regardless of which regimen was used for the primary series.
- If immunization is not initiated (i.e., child is behind) **until age 15–59 months**, then there is catch-up (1 dose), but **not given after age 5 years in normal children**
- Invasive disease does not confirm immunity; patients still require vaccines if age appropriate, i.e., age <5 years.

Pneumococcal Vaccines

- Pneumococcal conjugate vaccine (PCV13),
  - Purified polysaccharides of 13 serotypes conjugated to diphtheria protein
  - Routine administration as a **4-dose series for all children age 15 months and younger**
  - If no dose given yet between age 15–59 months, then there are catch-up doses
- 23-valent pneumococcal polysaccharide vaccine (PS23)—**given as additional protection to the PCV13 in some high-risk children (e.g., functional/anatomic asplenia) age >2 years**

Varicella

- Recommended at **age 12 months or older for healthy people who have not had varicella illness, with second dose at age 4–6 years**
- **Catch-up dosing:** both doses should be given for proper immunity
- May still have breakthrough varicella; milder than unimmunized, rarely spreads
- Has been associated with the development of herpes zoster after immunization (rare)
- Most people age >18 years, even without a reliable history of varicella infection, will still be immune.

MMR

- Live attenuated vaccine: issues as above for varicella
- First dose given at **age 12–15 months**
- Second dose given at **preschool age, 4–6 years**
- Catch-up with 2 doses

Hepatitis A Vaccine

- Recommended for all children age >1 year (**12–23 months**)
- **Two doses, 6 months apart**
- Also recommended routinely for chronic liver disease patients, homosexual and bisexual men, users of illegal drugs, patients with clotting-factor disorders, and those at risk of occupational exposure
- Can give with other vaccines

Meningococcal Conjugate Vaccine (MCV4)

Note

MPSV4 is the older, pure polysaccharide vaccine, while MCV4 is the newer, conjugated vaccine.

- Administer MCV4 to
    - All children at **the age 11–12 visit and booster at age 16**
    - **All college freshmen living in dormitories, if not vaccinated**
    - There is now a vaccine for **serotype B** to be used for high risk patients and during outbreaks (status post concurrent type B outbreaks at Princeton and UC Santa Barbara)

Influenza Vaccine

- Inactivated influenza vaccine (typical flu shot)
    - Administered intramuscularly
    - Caution in egg allergy (it has been found that most patients with no documented severe allergy to eggs can safely receive the vaccine; **appropriate cautions should be taken** and they should be watched in the medical setting for at least 30 minutes thereafter)
    - Given annually during flu season for children greater than 6 months of age (A strains, B strains, and H_1N_1)
- Live influenza vaccine
    - Administered intranasally
    - Contraindicated in the immunocompromised
    - Given *only to healthy people 2–49 years of age* who are not pregnant and do not have certain health conditions

Rotavirus Vaccine

- Oral live attenuated vaccine
- Given at ages 2, 4, 6 months
- Essentially no catch-up if behind (no dose after age 8 months)
- Safe, highly effective (no intussusception; M and M from disease reduced significantly)

Human Papilloma Virus Vaccine (HPV)

- Quadrivalent vaccine (6, 11, 16, 18) or bivalent vaccine (16, 18) to girls at the age 11-12 visit (through age 26) for cervical cancer prevention
- Quadrivalent vaccine (6, 11, 16, 18) to boys age 11–12; for genital warts caused by HPV 6,11.
- Can give in both males and females as early as age 9.
- 3 doses
    - Now 9-valent in both girls (9-26) and boys (9-15): 6,11 (genital warts), 16, 18, 31, 33, 45, 52, 58 (cervical cancer prevention)
    - Precancerous lesions (all 9) including anal intraepithelial neoplasia
    - Anal cancer (16,18,31,33,45,52,58)
- Doses 2 and 3: give at 2 months and then 6 months after first

Recommended immunization schedule for persons aged 0 through 18 years – United States, 2016.

(FOR THOSE WHO FALL BEHIND OR START LATE, SEE THE CATCH-UP SCHEDULE).

These recommendations must be read with the footnotes that follow. For those who fall behind or start late, provide catch-up vaccination at the earliest opportunity as indicated by the green bars in Figure 1. To determine minimum intervals between doses, see the catch-up schedule. School entry and adolescent vaccine age groups are shaded.

Vaccine	Birth	1 mo	2 mos	4 mos	6 mos	9 mos	12 mos	15 mos	18 mos	19–23 mos	2-3 yrs	4-6 yrs	7-10 yrs	11-12 yrs	13–15 yrs	16–18 yrs
Hepatitis B[1] (HepB)	1st dose	←— 2nd dose —→			←———————————— 3rd dose ————————————→											
Rotavirus[2] (RV) RV1 (2-dose series); RV5 (3-dose series)			1st dose	2nd dose	See footnote 2											
Diphtheria, tetanus, & acellular pertussis[3] (DTaP: <7 yrs)			1st dose	2nd dose	3rd dose			←———— 4th dose ————→				5th dose				
Haemophilus influenzae type b[4] (Hib)			1st dose	2nd dose	See footnote 4		←— 3rd or 4th dose, See footnote 4 —→									
Pneumococcal conjugate[5] (PCV13)			1st dose	2nd dose	3rd dose		←— 4th dose —→									
Inactivated poliovirus[6] (IPV: <18 yrs)			1st dose	2nd dose	←———————————— 3rd dose ————————————→							4th dose				
Influenza[7] (IIV; LAIV)					←———— Annual vaccination (IIV only) 1 or 2 doses ————————→						Annual vaccination (LAIV or IIV) 1 or 2 doses			Annual vaccination (LAIV or IIV) 1 dose only		
Measles, mumps, rubella[8] (MMR)					See footnote 8		←— 1st dose —→					2nd dose				
Varicella[9] (VAR)							←— 1st dose —→					2nd dose				
Hepatitis A[10] (HepA)							←— 2-dose series, See footnote 10 —→									
Meningococcal[11] (Hib-Mer CY ≥ 6 weeks; MenACWY-D ≥9 mos; MenACWY-CRM ≥ 2 mos)			←———————————————————— See footnote 11 ————————————————————→											1st dose		Booster
Tetanus, diphtheria, & acellular pertussis[12] (Tdap: ≥7 yrs)														(Tdap)		
Human papillomavirus[13] (2vHPV: females only; 4vHPV, 9vHPV: males and females)														(3-dose series)		
Meningococcal B[11]														←———— See footnote 11 ————→		
Pneumococcal polysaccharide[5] (PPSV23)												←———————————— See footnote 5 ————————————→				

Legend:
- Range of recommended ages for all children
- Range of recommended ages for catch-up immunization
- Range of recommended ages for certain high-risk groups
- Range of recommended ages for non-high-risk groups that may receive vaccine, subject to individual clinical decision making
- No recommendation

This schedule includes recommendations in effect as of January 1, 2016. Any dose not administered at the recommended age should be administered at a subsequent visit, when indicated and feasible. The use of a combination vaccine generally is preferred over separate injections of its equivalent component vaccines. Vaccination providers should consult the relevant Advisory Committee on Immunization Practices (ACIP) statement for detailed recommendations, available online at http://www.cdc.gov/vaccines/hcp/acip-recs/index.html. Clinically significant adverse events that follow vaccination should be reported to the Vaccine Adverse Event Reporting System (VAERS) online (http://www.vaers.hhs.gov) or by telephone (800-822-7967). Suspected cases of vaccine-preventable diseases should be reported to the state or local health department. Additional information, including precautions and contraindications for vaccination, is available from CDC online (http://www.cdc.gov/vaccines/recs/vac-admin/contraindications.htm) or by telephone (800-CDC-INFO [800-232-4636]).

This schedule is approved by the Advisory Committee on Immunization Practices (http://www.cdc.gov/vaccines/acip), the American Academy of Pediatrics (http://www.aap.org), the American Academy of Family Physicians (http://www.aafp.org), and the American College of Obstetricians and Gynecologists (http://www.acog.org).

NOTE: The above recommendations must be read along with the footnotes of this schedule.

For more details and specific footnotes, go to cdc.gov/ vaccines.

Child Abuse and Neglect 7

Learning Objectives

❏ Define physical, sexual, and psychological abuse

❏ Describe the epidemiology of child abuse

INTRODUCTION

Table 7-1. Scope of Child Abuse and Neglect

Physical		Psychological	
Abuse	Neglect	Abuse	Neglect
Fractures	Food	Terrorizing	Love
Bruises	Clothing	Putting down	Support
Burns	Schooling	Comparing	Stimulation
	Medical care	Insulting	Recognition
	Safety		

- Definitions
  - **Child maltreatment**—abusive actions or acts of commission and lack of action, or acts of omission that result in morbidity or death
  - **Physical abuse**—intentional injuries to a child by a caregiver that result in bruises, burns, fractures, lacerations, punctures, or organ damage; also may be accompanied by short- or long-term emotional consequences
  - **Psychological maltreatment**—intentional verbal or behavioral acts or omissions that result in adverse emotional consequences—spurning, exploiting/corrupting, withholding emotional responsiveness, isolating, terrorizing
  - **Sexual abuse**—any act intended for sexual gratification of an adult
  - **Factitious disorder**—intentionally giving poisons or toxins, or any other deceptive action to simulate a disorder
- Consequences
  - Failure-to-thrive (FTT)—nutritional neglect is most common cause of underweight infants (>50% of all cases of FTT)
  - Developmental delay
  - Learning disabilities

Note

Physicians and other care providers to children are required by law in all 50 states to report suspected abuse and neglect.

- Affords lawsuit protection to those who report in good faith
- Allows for all clinical and lab evaluation and documentation without parents' permission
- Failure to report may result in penalties
- Failure to report may result in malpractice claims for damages

– Physical disabilities

– Death

Epidemiology

- Higher likelihood of abuse with:
  - Caregivers have history of abuse or violence
  - Young parental age
  - Closely spaced pregnancies
  - Lower socioeconomic status
  - On military bases
  - Spousal abuse
  - Substance abuse
  - Single parent (mother)
  - Mentally retarded child
  - High stress level
  - Preterm, low-birth-weight infants

PHYSICAL ABUSE

A 2-year-old boy presents to the emergency department with a skull fracture that the mother states the child acquired after falling from a sofa onto a carpeted floor. During the physical examination the child is alert. He is noted to have old bruising on the buttocks and back, as well as a cigarette burn on his palm. The mother states that the child "falls a lot" and is always touching things he should not.

Diagnosis

- When to suspect
  - Injury is unexplained or implausible
  - Injury is incompatible with the history given or with child's level of development
  - There are no reports of death or serious brain injury from witnessed falls <10 feet.

Clinical Findings

Bruises

- Most common
- Accidental—thin, leading surfaces overlying bone edges (e.g., shins)
- Nonaccidental—buttocks, genitals, back, back of hands, thoraco-abdominal
- Shape of injury suggests object used—suspect with bilateral, symmetric, or geometric injuries
- Staging–**bruises in various stages are not compatible with a single event**
- Consider cultural issues, e.g., coining, cupping

> **Note**
>
> - Certainty is **not** required to file report to Child Protective Services (CPS).
> - However, one must determine whether parents have an understanding of disease processes and intellectual, emotional, economic, and physical resources to provide for child.

> **Note**
>
> Battered child syndrome is suggested by bruises, scars, internal organ damage, and fractures in various stages of healing.

Fractures

- Wrenching or pulling an extremity → corner **chip** or **bucket handle fracture** of metaphysis
- Inflicted fracture of bone shaft → more likely are **spiral fractures** from twisting rather than transverse from impact
- **A spiral fracture of the femur before child can walk independently has usually been inflicted by someone else.**
- Accidental impact rarely causes rib fractures or retinal hemorrhages in children.
- Highly specific for abuse
  - Rib fractures in infants
  - Fractures of different stages of healing
  - Bilateral fractures
  - Complex skull fracture

Burns

- Cigarette burns → circular, punched-out lesions of uniform size
- Immersion burns (most common in infants)
  - Glove-stocking pattern of extremity
  - Dipping into bathtub water:
    - Demarcation is uniform and distinct
    - Flexion creases spared
    - No splash burns
    - Hands and feet spared
    - **Incompatible with falling into tub or turning on hot water while in tub**

Intentional head trauma

- Most common cause of death
- **Consider when injured infant presents with coma, convulsions, apnea, increased ICP**
- A subdural hemorrhage in which there are no scalp marks or skull fracture is possibly from a hand blow.
- Retinal hemorrhages
- Shaking—acceleration-deceleration; may have no external marks; 85% associated with retinal hemorrhage

Note

Differential Diagnosis
With osteogenesis imperfecta or severe osteomalacia, there is an increased incidence of pathologic fractures, **but** they are rarely of the metaphysis.

Note

Always obtain a CT scan for intracranial bleeding and an eye exam for retinal hemorrhages.

Intra-abdominal injuries

- Impacts
- Recurrent vomiting, abdominal distension, absent bowel sounds, localized tenderness, shock
- If struck with fist → row of 3–4 teardrop-shaped, 1-cm bruises in a slight curve
- May rupture liver or spleen
- Laceration of small intestine at sites of ligamental support
- Intramural hematoma → temporary obstruction
- Free air

Laboratory Studies

- **Skeletal survey when you suspect abuse in child age <2 years; in child >2 years, appropriate film area of injury, complete survey not usually required**
- If infant is severely injured **despite** absence of CNS findings
  - Head CT scan
  - ± MRI
  - Ophthalmologic examination
- If abdominal trauma
  - Urine and stool for blood
  - Liver and pancreatic enzymes
  - Abdominal CT scan
- For any bleeding, bruises: PT, PTT, platelets, bleeding time, INR

Management. The first step is always to institute **prompt medical, surgical, or psychological treatment.**

- Consider separating child from caregiver in exam area.
- Report any child **suspected** of being abused or neglected to CPS; caseworker confers with M.D.
- Law enforcement agency performs forensics, interviews suspects, and if criminal act has taken place, informs prosecutor (state by state)
- Initial action includes a phone report, then, in most states,, a written report is required within 48 hours
- **Hospitalization is required if**
  - **Medical condition requires it**
  - **Diagnosis is unclear**
  - **There is no alternative safe place**
  - **Parents refuse hospitalization/treatment; M.D. must get emergency court order**
- M.D. should explain to parents
  - Why an inflicted injury is suspected
  - That M.D. is legally obligated to report
  - That referral is made to protect the child
  - That family will be provided with services
  - That a CPS worker and law enforcement officer will be involved
- Court ultimately decides guilt and disposition

Prognosis. The earlier the age of abuse, the greater the risk of mortality.

SEXUAL ABUSE

A 3-year-old girl presents with green vaginal discharge. Microscopic examination of the discharge revealed gram-negative intracellular diplococci.

- Epidemiology
  - Least common offender is a stranger
  - Most common reported abuse is that of daughters by fathers and stepfathers
  - **Most common overall is brother-sister incest**
  - Violence is not common but increases with age and size of victim
  - More likely to occur as a single incident with a stranger
- Clinical findings—sexual abuse should be **considered as a possible cause** if presenting with
  - Vaginal, penile, or rectal pain, discharge, bruising, erythema, or bleeding
  - Chronic dysuria, enuresis, constipation, or encopresis
  - **Any STDs in prepubertal child**
- Diagnosis
  - Test for pregnancy
  - Test for STDs
  - Test for syphilis, HIV, gonorrhea, hepatitis B
- Management:
  - Police and CPS notification
  - Psychiatric support
  - Foster care placement
  - Antibiotics, pregnancy (postmenarche in midcycle within 72 hours)

Note

Condyloma appearing after age 3 and *Trichomonas vaginalis* are probable diagnoses.

HSV-1 and nonvenereal warts may be autoinoculated.

Respiratory Disease 8

Learning Objectives

❑ Demonstrate understanding of upper airway obstruction from foreign bodies, congenital anomalies, and acute inflammatory upper airway obstruction

❑ Answer questions about inflammatory and infectious disorders of the small airways

❑ Describe the epidemiology and treatment of cystic fibrosis

❑ Recognize risk factors and presentation of sudden infant death syndrome

ACUTE INFLAMMATORY UPPER AIRWAY OBSTRUCTION

Croup

A 12-month-old child is brought to your office because of a barky cough. The mother states that over the past 3 days the child has developed a runny nose, fever, and cough. The symptoms are getting worse, and the child seems to have difficulty breathing. He sounds like a seal when he coughs.

- Infective agents—parainfluenza types 1, 2, 3
- Age 3 months–5 years; most common in winter; recurrences decrease with increasing growth of airway
- Inflammation of subglottis
- Signs and symptoms/examination—upper respiratory infection 1–3 days, then **barking cough, hoarseness, inspiratory stridor**; worse at night, gradual resolution over 1 week
- Complications—hypoxia only when obstruction is complete
- Diagnosis—**clinical, x-ray not needed (steeple sign if an x-ray is performed)**
- Treatment is basically supportive, but for more severe cases:
  - Nebulized epinephrine, followed by
  - Corticosteroids

Epiglottitis

A 2-year-old child presents to the emergency center with her parents because of high fever and difficulty swallowing. The parents state that the child had been in her usual state of health but awoke with fever of 40°C (104°F), a hoarse voice, and difficulty swallowing. On physical examination, the patient is sitting in a tripod position. She is drooling, has inspiratory stridor, nasal flaring, and retractions of the suprasternal notch and supraclavicular and intercostal spaces.

- Infective agents
    - *Haemophilus influenzae* type B (HiB) no longer number one (vaccine success)
    - Now combination of *Streptococcus pyogenes, Streptococcus pneumoniae, Staphylococcus aureus, Mycoplasma*
    - Risk factor—adult or unimmunized child
- Inflammation of epiglottis and supraglottis
- Signs and symptoms/examination—dramatic acute onset
    - High fever, sore throat, dyspnea, and rapidly progressing obstruction
    - **Toxic-appearing**, difficulty swallowing, drooling, **sniffing-position**
    - **Stridor is a late finding (near-complete obstruction)**
- Complications—complete airway obstruction and death
- Diagnosis
    - **Clinical first** (do nothing to upset child), controlled visualization (laryngoscopy) of **cherry-red, swollen epiglottis; x-ray not needed (thumb sign if x-ray is performed)** followed by immediate intubation
- Treatment
    - **Establish patent airway** (intubate)
    - Antibiotics to cover staphylococci, HiB, and resistant strep (antistaphylococcal plus third-generation cephalosporin)

Table 8-1. Croup, and, Epiglottitis

Feature	Croup	Epiglottitis
Etiology	• Parainfluenza 1,2,3	• *S. aureus* • *S. pneumonia, S. pyogenes* • *H. influenza* type B
Age	• Preschool	• Toddler-young school age
Timing	• Cool months	• Year round
Diagnosis Key Words	• Barking cough • Inspiratory stridor • If the patient gets worse: Inspiratory stridor ↓ Expiratory stridor (biphasic stridor) ↓ Stridor at rest	• Acute onset • Extremely sore throat • Cannot swallow • High fever • Sniffing position • Drooling • Inspiratory stridor later
Best Initial Test	• Clinical Dx • CXR not needed-but shows steeple sign	• Laryngoscopy
Most Accurate Test	• PCR for virus • Not needed clinically	• C and S from tracheal aspirate
Best Initial Treatment	• None or nebulized epinephrine if severe	• Airway (intubation)

Definitive Treatment (If Needed)	• Parenteral steroid
	  – Most common-single dose IM Dexamethasone →
	  – Observation
		• Airway (tracheostomy if needed) + broad-spectrum antibiotics
		• Then per sensitivities

CONGENITAL ANOMALIES OF THE LARYNX

Laryngomalacia

- Most common laryngeal airway anomaly and is the **most frequent cause of stridor in infants and children**.
- Collapse of supraglottic structures inward during inspiration stridor; less in prone position
- Starts in first 2 weeks of life, and symptoms increase up to 6 months of life; typically exacerbated by any exertion
- Diagnosis—Clinical suspicion is confirmed with **laryngoscopy**, bronchoscopy (for associated anomalies).
- Treatment—with most, supportive care; if significant, surgery (supraglottoplasty may prevent tracheostomy)

Congenital Subglottic Stenosis

- Second most common cause of stridor
- Common presentation—recurrent/persistent croup, i.e., stridor (no difference supine vs. prone position)
- Diagnosis—airway x-rays; confirm with laryngoscopy
- Treatment—surgery (cricoid split or reconstruction), may avoid tracheostomy

Vocal Cord Paralysis

- Third most common cause of stridor
- Often associated with meningomyelocele, Chiari malformation, hydrocephalus
- May be acquired after surgery from congenital heart defects or tracheoesophageal fistula (TEF) repair
- Bilateral—airway obstruction, high-pitched inspiratory stridor
- Unilateral—aspiration, cough, choking, weak cry and breathing
- Diagnosis—**flexible bronchoscopy**
- Treatment—usually resolves in 6–12 months; may require temporary tracheostomy

AIRWAY FOREIGN BODY

A toddler presents to the emergency center after choking on some coins. The child's mother believes that the child swallowed a quarter. On physical examination, the patient is noted to be drooling and in moderate respiratory distress. There are decreased breath sounds on the right with intercostal retractions.

Note

Larynx is the most common site of foreign body aspiration in children age <1 year.

In children age >1 year, think trachea or right mainstem bronchus.

- Most seen in children age 3–4 years
- Most common foreign body is peanuts
- Highly suggested if symptoms are *acute* choking, coughing, wheezing; often a witnessed event
- Clinical—depends on location
  - Sudden onset of respiratory distress
  - Cough, hoarseness, shortness of breath
  - Wheezing ((asymmetric) and decreased breath sounds (asymmetric))
- Complications—obstruction, erosion, infection (fever, cough, pneumonia, hemoptysis, atelectasis)
- Diagnosis—Chest x-ray reveals airtrapping (ball-valve mechanism). **Bronchoscopy** for definite diagnosis.
- Therapy—removal by **rigid bronchoscopy**

INFLAMMATORY DISORDERS OF THE SMALL AIRWAYS

Bronchiolitis

A 6-month-old infant presents to the physician with a 3-day history of upper respiratory tract infection, wheezy cough, and dyspnea. On physical examination, the patient has a temperature of 39°C (102°F), respirations of 60 breaths/min, nasal flaring, and accessory muscle usage. The patient appears to be air hungry, and the oxygen saturation is 92%.

- Infective agents—**respiratory syncytial virus** (**RSV**) (50%), parainfluenza, adenovirus, *Mycoplasma*, other viruses
- Typical age—almost all children infected by age <2 years, most severe at age 1–2 months in winter months.
- Inflammation of the small airways (inflammatory obstruction: edema, mucus, and cellular debris) → (bilateral) obstruction → air-trapping and overinflation
- Clinical presentation
  - Signs and symptoms:
    - Mild URI (often from household contact), decreased appetite and fever, irritability, paroxysmal wheezy cough, dyspnea, and tachypnea
    - **Apnea** may be more prominent early in young infants.
  - Examination:
    - Wheezing, increased work of breathing, fine crackles, prolonged expiratory phase
    - Lasts average of 12 days (worse in first 2–3 days)
- Complications—bacterial superinfection, respiratory insufficiency and failure (worse in infants with small airways and decreased lung function)
- Diagnosis
  - Clinical
  - Chest x-ray (not routine)—hyperinflation with patchy atelectasis (may look like early pneumonia)
  - Immunofluorescence of nasopharyngeal swab (not routine); PCR
- Treatment
  - Supportive care; hospitalize if respiratory distress; may give trial of hypertonic saline nebulization
  - **No steroids**
  - Ribavirin not routinely used; may prevent need for mechanical ventilation in severe cases
- Prevention—monoclonal antibody to RSV F protein (preferred: palivizumab) in **high-risk patients only**

PNEUMONIA

A 3-year-old child presents to the physician with a temperature of 40°C (104°F), tachypnea, and a wet cough. The patient's sibling has similar symptoms. The child attends daycare but has no history of travel or pet exposure. The child has a decreased appetite but is able to take fluids and has good urine output. Immunizations are up to date.

- Definition—inflammation of the lung parenchyma
- Epidemiology
  - **Viruses are predominant cause in infants and children age <5 years**
    ◦ Major pathogen—**RSV**
    ◦ Others—parainfluenza, influenza, adenovirus
    ◦ More in fall and winter
  - **Nonviral causes** more common in **children >5 years**
    ◦ Most—***M. pneumoniae* and *C. pneumoniae*** (genus has been changed to *Chlamydophila*; but remains *Chlamydia* for trachomatis)
    ◦ *S. pneumoniae* most common with focal infiltrate in children of all ages
    ◦ Others in normal children—*S. pyogenes* and *S. aureus* (no longer HiB)

Table 8-2. Clinical Findings in Viral Versus Bacterial Pneumonia

	Viral	Bacterial
Temperature	↑	↑↑↑
Upper respiratory infection	++	—
Toxicity	+	+++
Rales	Scattered	Localized
WBC	Normal to ↓	↑↑↑
Chest x-ray	Streaking, patchy	Lobar
Diagnosis	Nasopharyngeal washings	Blood culture, transtracheal aspirate (rarely done)

- Clinical findings
  - Viral:
    ◦ Usually several days of URI symptoms; low-grade fever
    ◦ Most consistent manifestation is tachypnea
    ◦ If severe—cyanosis, respiratory fatigue
    ◦ Examination—scattered crackles and wheezing
    ◦ **Difficult to localize source in young children with hyper-resonant chests; difficult to clinically distinguish viral versus nonviral**

- Bacterial pneumonia:
  - **Sudden shaking chills with high fever, acute onset**
  - Significant cough and chest pain
  - Tachypnea; productive cough
  - Splinting on affected side—minimize pleuritic pain
  - Examination—diminished breath sounds, localized crackles, rhonchi early; with increasing consolidation, **markedly diminished breath sounds and dullness to percussion**
- *Chlamydia trachomatis* pneumonia:
  - No fever or wheezing (serves to distinguish from RSV)
  - **1–3 months of age**, with insidious onset
  - May or may not have conjunctivitis at birth
  - Mild interstitial chest x-ray findings
  - **Staccato cough**
  - **Peripheral eosinophilia**
- *Chlamydophila pneumoniae* and *mycoplasma pneumoniae*
  - Cannot clinically distinguish
  - Atypical, insidious pneumonia; constitutional symptoms
  - **Bronchopneumonia**; gradual onset of constitutional symptoms with persistence of cough and hoarseness; coryza is unusual (usually viral)
  - Cough worsens with dyspnea over 2 weeks, then gradual improvement over next 2 weeks; becomes more productive; **rales** are most consistent finding (basilar)
- Diagnosis
  - Chest x-ray confirms diagnosis:
    - Viral—**hyperinflation with bilateral interstitial infiltrates and peribronchial cuffing**
    - Pneumococcal—**confluent lobar consolidation**
    - *Mycoplasma*—unilateral or bilateral lower-lobe interstitial pneumonia; **looks worse than presentation**
    - *Chlamydia*—interstitial pneumonia or lobar; as with *Mycoplasma*, chest x-ray often looks worse than presentation
  - White blood cells:
    - Viral—usually <20,000/mm^3 with lymphocyte predominance
    - Bacterial—usually 15,000–40,000/mm^3 with mostly granulocytes
    - *Chlamydia*—**eosinophilia**
  - Definitive diagnosis:
    - Viral— isolation of virus or detection of antigens in respiratory tract secretions; (usually requires 5–10 days); rapid reagents available for RSV, parainfluenza, influenza, and adenovirus
    - Bacterial—isolation of organism from blood (positive in only 10–30% of children with *S. pneumoniae*), pleural fluid, or lung; **sputum cultures are of no value in children.** For mycoplasma get IgM titers.

- Treatment
  - Based on presumptive cause and clinical appearance
  - Hospitalized—parenteral cefuroxime (if *S. aureus* suspected, add vancomycin or clindamycin)
  - **If suspect viral (outpatient, mild)—may withhold treatment *if* mild and no respiratory distress. Up to 30% may have coexisting bacterial pathogens**; deterioration should signal possible secondary bacterial infection and should start empiric treatment.
  - *Chlamydophila* or *Mycoplasma*—**erythromycin** or other macrolide

Table 8-3. Pneumonia

Feature	Bacterial	Viral	C. trachomatis	M. pneumoniae or C. pneumonia
Etiology	• *S. pneumoniae* • *HIB* • *S. aureus*	• *RSV* • *Parainfluenza* • *Influenza* • *Adenovirus*	*C. Trachomatis*	• *M. Pneumoniae* • *C. Pneumonia*
Age	• Any age • Most common reason for lobar is *S. pneumoniae*	Most common form <5 years	Age 1–3 months	Most common form age >5 years
Timing	More in cold months	Cold months	All year	All year; more in winter
Diagnosis Key Words	• Acute • Severe • Productive cough • Dyspnea • High fever • Chest pain • Rhonchi • Rales • Decreased breath sounds • May have empyema	• Insidious • Often worsening URI • Lower temperature • Wheeze • Cough • Mild dyspnea	• May have had conjunctivitis as newborn • Afebrile • No wheeze • Staccato cough	• Insidious • URI symptoms with persistence of cough worsening over 2 weeks • Rales most consistent finding (lower lobe uni- or bilateral)
Best Initial Test	• CXR = lobar consolidation	• CXR = bronchopneumonia, interstitial • Hyperinflation with increased peribronchial markings	• CXR = mild interstitial	• CXR most unilateral lower lobe interstitial • Classically looks worse than symptoms
Most Accurate Test	• Sputum C and S (cannot rely on in child) • Blood culture • Pleural fluid culture	Respiratory secretions for viral or antigen isolation (would not do routinely)	Sputum PCR (but not needed = classic clinical diagnosis)	PCR of NP or throat swab (but not usually needed)
Best Initial Treatment and Definitive Treatment	• Admit for IV cefuroxime • Then change if needed based on C and S	• No treatment of viral pneumonia • If uncertain, give oral amoxicillin	Oral macrolide	Oral macrolide

CYSTIC FIBROSIS (CF)

A 3-year-old white child presents with rectal prolapse. She is noted to be in the less than 5th percentile for weight and height. The parents also note that she has a foul-smelling bulky stool each day that "floats." They also state that the child has developed a repetitive cough over the last few months.

- Most common life-limiting recessive trait among whites
- Major cause of severe chronic lung disease and most common cause of exocrine pancreatic deficiency in children
- Primary pathogenic feature is dysfunction of epithelialized surfaces; obstruction and infection of airways; maldigestion
- Genetics
    - **Autosomal recessive**; CF gene most prevalent among **northern and central Europeans**
    - All of the gene mutations occur at a single locus on long arm of **chromosome 7.**
    - Codes for CF transmembrane regulator (**CFTR**—ion channel and regulatory functions)
        ○ Expressed mostly on epithelial cells of airways, gastrointestinal tract, sweat glands, genitourinary (GU) system
        ○ Not all children with CF can be identified by DNA testing; may need to sequence CFTR gene
- Pathogenesis and pathology
    - Membranes of CF epithelial cells **unable to secrete Cl⁻** in response to cyclic adenosine monophosphate–mediated signals:
        ○ **Failure to clear mucous secretions**; paucity of water in mucous secretions
        ○ Increased salt content of sweat and other serous secretions
        ○ Manifestations:
            ▸ Bronchiolar obliteration, bronchiectasis (end-stage; severe destructive disease)
            ▸ Opacified paranasal sinuses
            ▸ Large nasal polyps
            ▸ Pancreatic dysfunction; fat and fat-soluble vitamin malabsorption
            ▸ Intestinal glands distended with mucous secretions; focal biliary cirrhosis
            ▸ Endocervitis
            ▸ Body and tail of epididymis, vas deferens, seminal vesicles obliterated or atretic in males
- Clinical presentation
    - Intestinal tract—usually first presentation:
        ○ 10% of newborns with **meconium ileus**
            ▸ X-ray shows dilated loops, air–fluid levels, "ground-glass" (bubbly appearance) material in lower central abdomen
            ▸ Gastrografin enema → reflux into ileum may clear; if not, then surgery
        ○ Most with malabsorption from pancreatic exocrine insufficiency → **frequent, bulky, greasy stools and failure-to-thrive.**

- ○ **Fat-soluble vitamin deficiency—ADEK**
- ○ Hepatobiliary—icterus, ascites, hepatomegaly, cholelithiasis, varices
- ○ Pancreas—increased incidence of diabetes mellitus, **acute pancreatitis**
- ○ **Rectal prolapse**—most in infants with steatorrhea, malnutrition, and cough
- – Respiratory tract:
  - ○ **Rate of progression of lung disease is chief determinant of mortality and morbidity**—early in life—nontypable *H. influenzae* and *S. aureus*, then colonization with *P. aeruginosa*, then later colonization with ***Burkholderia cepacia***: associated with rapid deterioration and death (end-stage)
  - ○ **Cough, purulent mucus**—early in first year, extensive bronchiolitis, then pulmonary function test (PFT) abnormalities, dyspnea; finally, cor pulmonale, respiratory failure, and death; high risk for pneumothorax
  - ○ Examination:
    - ▸ Increased A-P diameter
    - ▸ **Hyper-resonance**, rales, **expiratory wheezing**
    - ▸ **Clubbing**, cyanosis (late)
    - ▸ Sinuses almost always opacified
- – Genitourinary tract:
  - ○ Delayed sexual development
  - ○ Almost all males with **azoospermia**
  - ○ Increased incidence of hernia, hydrocele, undescended testes
  - ○ Females: **secondary amenorrhea**, cervicitis, **decreased fertility**
- – Sweat glands:
  - ○ Excessive loss of salt → salt depletion, especially with hot weather or gastroenteritis (serum–hypochloremic alkalosis)
  - ○ **Salty taste of skin**
- • Diagnosis
  - – *See* Table 8-4.

Table 8-4. Diagnosing CF

Any of the Following	*Plus* Any of the Following
• Typical clinical features	• Two increased sweat chlorides on 2 separate days
• History of a sibling with CF	• Identification of 2 CF mutations (homozygous)
• Positive newborn screen	• Increased nasal potential difference

- – Sweat test (**best test**):
  - ○ Difficult in first weeks of life
  - ○ Confirm positive results
  - ○ Diagnosis: >60 mEq/L
- – If sweat test is equivocal:
  - ○ Increased potential difference across nasal epithelium
  - ○ Pancreatic function—72-hour fecal fat collection, stool for trypsin, pancreozymin-secretin stimulation, serum immunoreactive trypsinogen ($\uparrow$ in neonates)

- X-rays:
  - Hyperinflation of chest
  - Nodular densities, patchy atelectasis, confluent infiltrates, hilar nodes
  - With progression—flattening of diaphragm, sternal bowing, narrow cardiac shadow; cysts, extensive bronchiectasis
- Pulmonary function tests:
  - By 5 years—**obstructive** pulmonary disease
  - Then **restrictive (fibrosis)**
- Microbiologic—finding in sputum of **S. aureus** first, followed by **P. aeruginosa** (mucoid forms) is **virtually diagnostic** (also *B. cepacia*, but is usually late finding)
- Genetic:
  - Antenatal diagnosis by mutational analysis in family previously identified by birth of child with CF
  - Test spouse of carrier with standard panel of probes
  - **Newborn screen**—determination of immunoreactive trypsinogen in blood spots and then **confirmation with sweat or DNA testing; does *not* improve pulmonary and therefore long-term outcome**

• Treatment
  - Clear airway secretions and control infections:
    - **Aerosol treatment; albuterol/saline**
    - Daily dose of **human recombinant DNAse (mucolytic)**
    - Chest physical therapy with postural drainage: 1–4 times per day
  - Antibiotics:
    - For acute infections (change in baseline condition)
    - Most frequent is *P. aeruginosa* (also non-typable *H. influenzae*, *S. aureus*, *B. cepacia*)
    - Must base choice on culture and sensitivity
    - Aerosolized antibiotics—**tobramycin**
  - Hospitalization:
    - Progressive despite intensive home measures
    - Typical 14-day treatment
    - Two-drug regimens to cover pseudomonas, e.g., **piperacillin plus tobramycin or ceftazidime**
  - Nutritional: **pancreatic enzyme replacement with meals/snacks; vitamin supplementation (ADEK)**
  - **Adequate fluid replacement when exercising or hot weather**

SUDDEN INFANT DEATH SYNDROME (SIDS)

A 2-month-old term infant born with no complications via spontaneous vaginal delivery is brought to the emergency center via ambulance with CPR in progress. According to the mother, the patient was in his usual state of good health until 4 A.M. when she found him cyanotic and not breathing. At midnight the infant was fed 4 ounces of formula without any difficulty and then placed to sleep in a crib. At 4 A.M. the mother returned and found the child unresponsive. She immediately called emergency medical services and began CPR. The child was pronounced dead on arrival to the emergency department.

- **Definition**—sudden death of an infant, unexplained by history or by thorough postmortem examination including autopsy, investigation of death scene, and review of medical history; recently, new nomenclature is **Sudden Unexplained Infant Death Syndrome** (SUIDS)
- Before 1992, incidence was constant at 1.4 in 1,000; then with **Back to Sleep** campaign, down to 0.45 in 1,000
- Differential diagnosis
  - Explained at autopsy: infections; congenital anomaly; unintentional injury; traumatic child abuse; other natural causes
  - Not explained: SIDS; **intentional suffocation**
- Pathology: no findings are pathognomonic and none are diagnostic (markers for pre-existing, chronic, low-grade asphyxia): **petechial hemorrhages**; pulmonary edema
- Environmental risk factors
  - Nonmodifiable:
    - Low socioeconomic status
    - African American and Native American
    - **Highest at 2–4 months** of age; most by 6 months
    - Highest in winter, midnight to 9 A.M.
    - Males > females
  - Modifiable:
    - Shorter interpregnancy interval
    - Less prenatal care
    - Low birth weight, preterm, intrauterine growth retardation
    - **Maternal smoking**
    - **Postnatal smoking**
- **Sleep environment**
  - **Higher incidence related to prone sleeping**
  - **Supine position now better than side-lying**
  - No increased problems in supine, i.e., aspiration
  - Higher incidence with **soft bedding/surfaces**
  - Higher incidence with **overheating**
  - Pacifier shown to consistently decrease risk

- • Other risk factors
    - – Episode of an apparent life-threatening event (ALTE); recently, new nomenclature for ALTE is **Brief Resolved Unexplained Episode** (BRUE)
    - – Subsequent sibling of SIDS victim
    - – Prematurity—inverse with gestational age and birth weight
- • **Home monitors do not decrease risk.**
- • Reducing risk
    - – **Supine while asleep**
    - – Use crib that meets federal safety standards
    - – No soft surfaces (sofas, waterbeds, etc.)
    - – No soft materials in sleep environment
    - – No bed-sharing
    - – Avoid overheating and overbundling
    - – Use prone position only while infant is awake and observed
    - – No recommendation for home monitoring for this purpose
    - – Expand national Back to Sleep campaign (up to 25% of infants still sleep prone).

Allergy and Asthma   9

Learning Objectives

❏   Apply knowledge of allergies and asthma to diagnose and describe treatment options

ALLERGIES

Allergic Rhinitis

- Generally established by age 6 years
- Increased risk—early introduction of formula (versus breast milk) or solids, mother smoking before child is 1 year old, heavy exposure to indoor allergens
- Most perennial or mixed; increased symptoms with greater exposure
- **Diagnosis suggested by typical symptoms in absence of URI or structural abnormality (nasal congestion/pruritus, worse at night with snoring, mouth-breathing; watery, itchy eyes; postnasal drip with cough; possible wheezing; headache)**
- Specific behaviors
  - Allergic salute (rhinorrhea and nasal pruritus) → nasal crease
  - Vigorous grinding of eyes with thumb and side of fist
- History of symptoms
  - Timing and duration (seasonal versus perennial)
  - Exposures/settings in which symptoms occur
  - Family history of allergic disease (atopy, asthma)
  - Food allergies more common (nuts, seafood) in young children (then skin, gastrointestinal, and, less often, respiratory)
- Physical examination
  - **Allergic shiners** (venous stasis)—blue-gray-purple beneath lower eyelids; often with **Dennie lines**—prominent symmetric skin folds
  - Conjunctival injection, **chemosis** (edema), stringy discharge, "cobblestoning" of tarsal conjunctiva
  - **Transverse nasal crease (from allergic salute)**
  - **Pale nasal mucosa**, thin and clear secretions, **turbinate hypertrophy**, polyps
  - Postnasal drip (posterior pharynx)
  - Otitis media with effusion is common

- Differential diagnosis
  - **Nonallergic inflammatory rhinitis (no IgE antibodies)**
  - **Vasomotor rhinitis (from physical stimuli)**
  - **Nasal polyps (think of CF)**
  - **Septal deviation**
  - **Overuse of topical vasoconstrictors**
  - Rare: neoplasms; vasculitides; granulomatous disorders (Wegener)
- Laboratory evaluation (no initial routine labs; clinical DX)
  - In vitro:
    - Peripheral eosinophilia
    - Eosinophils in nasal and bronchial secretions; **more sensitive than blood eosinophils**
    - Increased serum IgE
    - IgE-specific allergen in blood draw (**advantages** are safety and the results will be uninfluenced by skin disease/medications, while major **disadvantages** are its expense and less sensitivity); best use is for extensive dermatitis and for medications that interfere with mast cell degranulation, have high risk for anaphylaxis, or cannot cooperate with skin tests
  - In vivo—**skin test (best):**
    - Use appropriate allergens for geographic area plus indoor allergens.
    - May not be positive before two seasons
- Treatment—environmental control plus removal of allergen is **most effective method**
  - Avoidance of biggest triggers—house dust mite, cat, cockroach
  - Dehumidifiers, HEPA-filtered vacuuming, carpet removal, pillow and mattress encasement
  - Remove pets
  - No smoking
  - No wood-burning stoves/fireplaces
- Pharmacologic control
  - **Antihistamines (first-line therapy):**
    - First generation—diphenhydramine, chlorpheniramine, brompheniramine; cross blood-brain barrier—sedating
    - **Second generation (cetirizine, fexofenadine, loratadine)**—nonsedating (**now preferred drugs**); easier dosing
    - **Oral antihistamines are more effective than cromolyn but significantly less than intranasal steroids; efficacy ↑ when combined with an intranasal steroid**
  - Intranasal corticosteroids—**most effective medication, but not first-line:**
    - Effective for all symptoms
    - Add to antihistamine if symptoms are more severe
  - Leukotriene-receptor antagonists
  - Chromones—cromolyn and nedocromil sodium:
    - Least effective
    - Very safe with prolonged use
    - Best for preventing an unavoidable allergen

Note

Differential Diagnosis of Eosinophilia

- Neoplasms
- Asthma/Allergy
- Addison disease
- Collagen Vascular Disorders
- Parasites

- Decongestants—(alpha-adrenergic → vasoconstriction)—topical forms (oxymetazoline, phenylephrine) significant **rebound** when discontinued.
- Epinephrine—alpha and beta adrenergic effects; **drug of choice for anaphylaxis**
- Immunotherapy:
  ○ Administer gradual increase in dose of allergen mixture → decreases or eliminates person's adverse response on subsequent natural exposure
  ○ **Major indication**—duration and severity of symptoms are disabling in spite of routine treatment (for at least two consecutive seasons). This, however, is the **treatment of choice for insect venom allergy**.
  ○ **Should not** be used for (lack of proof): atopic dermatitis, **food allergy,** latex allergy, urticaria, children age <3 years (too many systemic symptoms)
  ○ Need several years of treatment; expensive
- Complications of allergic rhinitis
  - Chronic sinusitis
  - Asthma
  - Eustachian tube obstruction → middle ear effusion
  - Tonsil/adenoid hypertrophy
  - Emotional/psychological problems

Insect Venom Allergy

- Etiology/pathophysiology—systemic allergic responses are IgE-mediated and are almost always due to stings from the order Hymenoptera (yellow jackets most notorious—aggressive, ground-dwelling, linger near food)
- Clinical presentation
  - Local—limited swelling/pain <1 day
  - Large local area—develop over hours to days; extensive swelling
  - Systemic—urticaria/angioedema, pruritus, **anaphylaxis**
  - Toxic—fever, malaise, emesis, nausea
  - Delayed/late response—serum sickness, nephrotic syndrome, vasculitis, neuritis, encephalitis
- Diagnosis—for biting/stinging insects, **must pursue skin testing**
- Treatment
  - Local—cold compresses, topical antipruritic, oral analgesic, systemic antihistamine; **remove stingers by scraping**
  - **If anaphylaxis—epinephrine pen**, ID bracelet, avoid attractants (e.g., perfumes)
  - **Indication for venom immune therapy—severe reaction with + skin tests (highly effective in decreasing risk)**

Food Reactions

- Clinical presentation
  - Most infants and young children **outgrow milk and egg allergy** (half in first 3 years); majority with nut or seafood allergies retain for life:
    ○ **Most food allergies are—egg, milk, peanuts, nuts, fish, soy, wheat, but any food may cause a food allergy.**

- ○ **Food allergic reactions are most common cause of anaphylaxis seen in emergency rooms**
- – With food allergies, there is an **IgE and/or a cell-mediated response.**
- – Manifestations:
  - ○ Skin—**urticaria/angioedema** and flushing, **atopic dermatitis;** 1/3 of children with atopic dermatitis have food allergies, but most common is acute urticaria/angioedema
  - ○ Gastrointestinal—oral pruritus, nausea, **vomiting, diarrhea, abdominal pain,** eosinophilic gastroenteritis **(often first symptoms to affect infants):** predominantly a **cell-mediated response, so standard allergy tests are of little value; food protein–induced enterocolitis/proctocolitis presents with bloody stool/diarrhea (most cow milk or soy protein allergies)**
  - ○ Respiratory—nasal congestion, rhinorrhea, sneezing, laryngeal edema, dyspnea, **wheezing, asthma**
  - ○ Cardiovascular—dysrhythmias, **hypotension**
- • Diagnosis
  - – Must establish the food and amount eaten, timing, and nature of reaction
  - – Skin tests, IgE-specific allergens are useful for IgE sensitization.
    - ○ A negative skin test excludes an IgE-mediated form, but because of cell-mediated responses, may need a **food elimination and challenge test** in a controlled environment **(best test)**
- • Treatment
  - – **Only validated treatment is elimination**
  - – **Epinephrine pens** for possible anaphylaxis

Urticaria and Angioedema

Causes:

- • Acute, IgE-mediated (duration ≤6 weeks)
  - – Activation of mast cells in skin
  - – Systemically absorbed allergen: food, drugs, stinging venoms; with allergy, penetrates skin → hives (urticaria)
- • Non IgE-mediated, but stimulation of mast cells
  - – **Radiocontrast agents**
  - – Viral agents (especially EBV, hepatitis B)
  - – Opiates, NSAIDs
- • Physical urticarias; environmental factors—temperature, pressure, stroking, vibration, light
- • Hereditary angioedema
  - – Autosomal dominant
  - – C1 esterase-inhibitor deficiency
  - – Recurrent episodes of nonpitting edema
- • Diagnosis mainly clinical; skin tests, IgE-specific allergens (blood)
- • Treatment
  - – Most respond to avoidance of trigger and oral antihistamine
  - – Severe—epinephrine, short-burst corticosteroids

- If H$_1$ antagonist alone does not work, **H$_1$ plus H$_2$** antagonists are effective; consider steroids
- For chronic refractory angioedema/urticaria → IVIg or plasmapheresis

Anaphylaxis

- Sudden release of active mediators with cutaneous, respiratory, cardiovascular, gastrointestinal symptoms
- Most common reasons
  - In hospital—**latex, antibiotics**, IVIg (intravenous immunoglobulin), radiocontrast agents
  - Out of hospital—food (**most common is peanuts**), insect sting, oral medications, idiopathic
- Presentation—reactions from ingested allergens are delayed (minutes to 2 hours); with injected allergen, reaction is immediate (more gastrointestinal symptoms)
- Treatment
  - What the patient should do immediately:
    ◦ **Injectable epinephrine**
    ◦ Oral liquid diphenhydramine
    ◦ Transport to ER
  - Medical:
    ◦ **Oxygen and airway management**
    ◦ Epinephrine IM (IV for severe hypotension); intravenous fluid expansion; H$_1$ antagonist; corticosteroids; nebulized, short-acting beta-2 agonist (with respiratory symptoms); H$_2$ antagonist (if oral allergen)

Atopic Dermatitis (Eczema)

- Epidemiology/pathophysiology
  - Interaction among genetic, environmental, and immunologic factors; familial with strong maternal influence
  - Majority develop allergic rhinitis and/or asthma
  - Most have increased eosinophils and IgE
- Clinical presentation
  - **Half start by age 1 year**; most by age 1 and 5 years; chronic or relapsing
  - Intense cutaneous reactivity and **pruritus**; worse at night; scratching induces lesions; becomes excoriated
  - Exacerbations with foods, inhalants, bacterial infection, decreased humidity, excessive sweating, irritants
  - Patterns for skin reactions:
    ◦ Acute: **erythematous papules, intensely pruritic, serous exudate and excoriation**
    ◦ Subacute—erythematous, excoriated, **scaling papules**
    ◦ Chronic—**lichenification** (thickening, darkening)

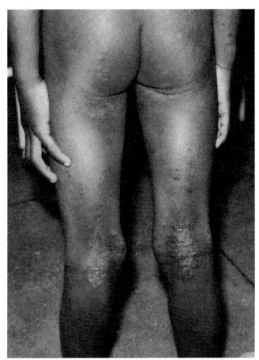

Courtesy of Tom D. Thacher, M.D.

Figure 9-1. Subacute and Chronic Atopic Dermatitis Most Commonly Affects the Flexural Surfaces of Joints

- – Distribution pattern:
  - ○ Infancy: **face, scalp, extensor** surfaces of extremities
  - ○ Older, long-standing disease: **flexural** aspects
  - ○ Often have remission with age, but skin left prone to itching and inflammation when exposed to irritants
- • Treatment
  - – Identify and eliminate causative factors
  - – **Cutaneous hydration**
    - ○ **Dry skin, especially in winter (xerosis)**
    - ○ Lukewarm soaking baths followed by application of occlusive emollient (hydrophilic ointments)
  - – **Topical corticosteroids**
    - ○ **Seven classes—the higher potency classes are not to be used on face or intertriginous areas and only for short periods**
    - ○ **Goal—emollients and low-potency steroids for maintenance**
  - – Topical immunomodulators; **tacrolimus** (calcineurin inhibitor):
    - ○ Inhibits activation of key cells
    - ○ Ointment safe and effective
    - ○ **Safe on face**
    - ○ Can use as young as age **2 years**

- Tar preparations
- Phototherapy—UV light
- Systemic: antihistamines (sedating at night; for pruritus); glucocorticoids; cyclosporine (refractory to all other treatment); interferon (if all else fails)
- Treat with antibiotics for bacterial superinfection
- Complications
  - Secondary bacterial infection, especially *S. aureus*; increased incidence of *T. rubrum*, *M. furfur*
  - Recurrent viral skin infections—**Kaposi varicelliform eruption (eczema herpeticum) most common**
  - Warts/molluscum contagiosum

Contact Dermatitis

- Irritant
  - Nonspecific injury to skin
  - Results from prolonged or repetitive contact with various substances (e.g., diaper rash)
- Allergic
  - **Delayed hypersensitivity reaction (type IV)**; provoked by antigen applied to skin surface
  - Intense itching; chronically can mimic atopic dermatitis
  - Distribution provides clue to diagnosis
  - Causes—jewelry (especially nickel), shoes, clothing, and plants (poison ivy)
- Diagnosis—clinical
- Treatment—supportive; eliminate contact with allergen; cool compresses

ASTHMA

A 6-year-old boy presents to his physician with end-expiratory wheezing scattered throughout the lung fields. He is noted to have nasal flaring, tachypnea, and intercostal retractions. These symptoms are triggered by changes in the weather. He has a family history of asthma and atopic dermatitis. He has never been intubated or admitted to the pediatric ICU. His last hospitalization for asthma was 6 months ago. He takes medication for asthma only when he starts to wheeze.

- Etiology/pathophysiology
  - Chronic inflammation of airways with episodic at least partially reversible airflow obstruction
    - Genetic and environmental factors: concomitant allergies (perennial in most), induced by common viral agents, tobacco smoke; cold, dry air; strong odors
    - Most with onset age <6 years; most resolve by late childhood
    - Two main patterns:
      - Early childhood triggered primarily by common **viral infections**
      - Chronic asthma associated with **allergies** (often into adulthood; atopic)

- - **Some risk factors for persistent asthma:** perennial allergies; atopic dermatitis, allergic rhinitis, food allergy; severe lower respiratory tract infections; wheezing other than with URIs (exercise, emotions); environmental tobacco smoke exposure; low birth weight
- Clinical presentation
  - **Diffuse wheezing, expiratory then inspiratory**
  - **Prolonged expiratory phase**
  - Decreased breath sounds
  - Rales/rhonchi → excess mucus and inflammatory exudate
  - Increased work of breathing
  - Exercise intolerance
- Diagnosis
  - **In children, neither lab tests nor provocation challenge tests are required for diagnosis; they may support the clinical diagnosis or may be used to follow the patient clinically.**
  - Lung function:
    - **Gold standard = spirometry during forced expiration.** $FEV_1/FVC <0.8 =$ airflow obstruction (the forced expiratory volume in 1 second adjusted to the full expiratory lung volume, i.e., the forced vital capacity) in children age ≥ 5 yrs
    - Bronchodilator response to inhaled beta-agonist—improvement in FEV_1 to >12%
    - Exercise challenge—worsening in FEV_1 of at least 15%
    - **Home tool—peak expiratory home monitoring (PEF);** A.M. and P.M. PEF for several weeks for practice and to establish personal best and to correlate to symptoms; based on personal best, divide PEFs into zones: green (80–100%), yellow (50–80%), red (<50%)
  - Radiology (no routine use):
    - **Hyperinflation—flattening of the diaphragms**
    - **Peribronchial thickening**
    - Use to identify other problems that may mimic asthma (e.g., aspiration with severe gastroesophageal reflux) and for complications during severe exacerbations (atelectasis, pneumonia, air leak)
- Treatment—based on asthma severity classification
  - Intermittent: symptoms ≤2 days/week and ≤2 nights/mo
    - No need for daily controller
  - Persistent (mild → moderate → severe) symptoms > intermittent
    - Need daily controller

Table 9-1. Severity Classification and Treatment (simplified from National Asthma Education and Prevention Program)

Class	Daytime Symptoms	Nighttime Symptoms	Treatment
Intermittent	≤2×/week	≤2×/month	Short-acting β, agonist PRN
Mild persistent	>2×/week	>2×/month	Inhaled steroids β agonist for, breakthrough
Moderate persistent	Daily	>1×/week	Inhaled steroids Long-acting β, agonist Short-acting β for, breakthrough Leukotrine-receptor antagonists
Severe persistent	Continual;, limited activities; frequent exacerbations	Frequent	High-dose inhaled steroid Long-acting β agonist Short-acting β agonist Systemic steroids Leukotrine-receptor antagonists

> **Note**
>
> With all asthma categories, a step-up, step-down dosing is typically used (high at first, then down to minimum necessary to prevent symptoms).

- Asthma medications
  - **Quick-relief medications**
    - Short-acting beta-2 agonists: **albuterol, levalbuterol** (nebulized only), terbutaline, metaproterenol (rapid onset, may last 4–6 hrs; **drug of choice for rescue and preventing exercise-induced asthma but inadequate control if need >1 canister/month**
    - Anticholinergics (much less potent than beta agonists): **ipratropium bromide**; mostly for added treatment of acute severe asthma in ED and hospital
    - Short-course systemic glucocorticoids: outpatient for moderate to severe flare-up, and prednisone 3–7 days; inpatient recommended with IV methylprednisolone IV
- Management of asthma exacerbations
  - Emergency department:
    - Monitor, **oxygen** as needed
    - Inhaled **albuterol** q 20 minutes for one hour—add **ipratropium** if no good response for second dose
    - **Corticosteroids PO or IV**
    - Can go home if sustained improvement with normal physical findings and **SaO_2 >92% after 4 hours in room air**; PEF ≥70% of personal best
    - Home on q 3–4 hour **MDI + 3–7-day oral steroid**
  - Hospital—**for moderate–severe flare-ups without improvement within 1–2 hours of initial acute treatment with PEF <70% of personal best or SaO_2 <92% on room air:**
    - **Oxygen**
    - Nebulized **albuterol** (very frequently or continuous)
    - Add **ipratropium** q 6 hours

> **Note**
>
> Older children can use a metered dose inhaler (MDI); younger children often need to do so with a spacer and face mask. Infants may need to have nebulized medications.

> **Note**
>
> Adjunct Treatment to Prevent Intubation and Ventilation
> - IV beta agonist
> - IV theophylline
> - Heliox (70:30 He:O_2); decreased airway resistance and clinical response in 20 min
> - IV $MgSO_4$— smooth-muscle relaxant; monitor BP every 10–15 min (risk of hypotension)

- Intravenous corticosteroids
  - May need intravenous fluids
  - Mechanical ventilation (rare)

Table 9-2. Bronchiolitis vs. Asthma

Feature	Bronchiolitis	Asthma
Etiology	Most RSV	Reversible bronchoconstriction with chronic inflammation
Age	Infants (especially <1 year)	Most start age <5 years
Timing	• Winter	• All year • Most with URI in winter
Diagnosis Key Words	• URI from another household contact • Getting worse • Fever • Tachypnea • Bilateral expiratory wheezing ± respiratory distress • Apnea	• Repeated episodes of expiratory wheezing • Chronic non-productive cough • Chest tightness • Respiratory distress • May have other atopic disease + family history • May occur primarily with URIs • Cannot make diagnosis of asthma for first-time wheezing in infant with fever (diagnosis is bronchiolitis)
Best Initial Test	• Clinical Dx • CXR only if severe and therefore possibility of secondary bacterial pneumonia	Worsening of FEV1/FVC with exercise and improvement with beta-agonist
Most Accurate Test	• NP rapid test or PCR for organism • ABG only for severe to evaluate possible need for ventilation	• Repeated episodes that improve with beta-agonist
Treatment	• Oxygen, if needed • Supportive Rx • May try nebulized hypertonic saline • Ribavirin in severe or worsening cases MAY prevent the need for intubation and ventilation	• Oxygen • Short-acting beta-agonist • Add oral steroid for acute attack • May need chronic maintenance Rx

Immune-Mediated Disease 10

Learning Objectives

❑ Explain information related to evaluation of suspected immune deficiency

❑ Categorize specific defects of immune deficiency

EVALUATION OF SUSPECTED IMMUNE DEFICIENCY

Table 10-1. Suspecting Immunodeficiency by Major Defect

	B-Cell	T-Cell	Complement	Neutrophil
Common organism	**Recurrent bacterial:** streptococci, staphylococci, *Haemophilus*, *Campylobacter*; ***Viral:*** *enteroviruses*; *Uncommon: giardia, cryptosporidia*	**Opportunistic organisms:** CMV, EBV, varicella, *Candida*, Pneumocystis jiroveci, mycobacteriwa	*Pneumococci, Neisseria*	**Bacteria:** Staphylococci, *Pseudomonas, Serratia, Klebsiella, Salmonella*; **Fungi:** *Candida, Aspergillus*
Age onset	5-7 months of age or later childhood to adult	Usually 2-6 months of age	Any age	Early onset
Infections	Most are **recurrent sinopulmonary infections and recurrent enteroviral meningitis**	**Mucocutaneous candidiasis;** pulmonary and GI infections	**Meningitis,** arthritis, septicemia, recurrent sinopulmonary infections	**Skin abscesses,** impetigo, cellulitis, **suppurative adenitis,** gingivitis, **oral ulcers,** osteomyelitis, internal organ abscesses
Other findings	**Autoimmunity, lymphoreticular malignancy**	**Chronic diarrhea and failure-to-thrive;** postvaccination dissemination - varicella, BCG; hypocalcemia in infancy; **graft-versus-host** from transplacental maternal engraftment or nonirradiated blood	Autoimmune disorders, vasculitis, glomerulonephritis, **angioedema**	**Prolonged attachment of umbilical cord,** poor wound healing, decreased signs of infection
Best initial test	**Screen with IgA→if low, measure IgG and IgM (quantitative immunoglobulins)**	Lymphocyte count (low)	Screen is total hemolytic complement (CH_{50})—will be depressed if any component is consumed	Neutrophil count
Other tests	Low antibody titers to specific antigens—isohemmaglutinins, vaccines	**Best cost-effective test for T-cell function –** *Candida* skin test	Identify mode of inheritance—all are autosomal except for properdin deficiency (X-linked)	Neutrophil respiratory burst after phorbol ester stimulation; most reliable now uses **rhodamine fluorescence (replaced the NBT test)**
Specific tests	Enumerate B-cells with **flow cytometry** (monoclonal antibodies to B-cell-specific CD antigens): B cell absent or present and number	Flow cytometry using monoclonal antibodies recognizing T-cell CD antigens (phytahemmaglutinin, concanavalin A, pokeweed mitogen)	Can easily measure C3 and C4 (hereditary angioedema); others require a research lab	Can identify leukocyte adhesion deficiencies with flow cytometric assays of lymphocytes and neutrophils (CD18, CD11, CD15)

Note: For each, the **most accurate test** is **molecular genetic diagnosis.**

SPECIFIC DEFECTS

Defects of Antibody Production

X-linked (Bruton) agammaglobulinemia

X-linked (Bruton) agammaglobulinemia (XLA) is a profound **defect in B-cell development** which leads to an absence of circulating B cells and thus leads to severe hypogammaglobulinemia **with small-to-absent tonsils and no palpable lymph nodes.**

- **Genetics:** >500 known mutations of the Btk gene (Bruton tyrosine kinase), which is necessary for pre-B-cell expansion and maturation; long arm of **X-chromosome**
- **Clinical findings: boys with pyogenic sinopulmonary infections**
- **Diagnosis:** clinical presentation + **lymphoid hypoplasia on exam; all immunoglobulins severely depressed**; flow cytometry shows absence of circulating B-cells; gene sequencing for specific mutation
- **Treatment:** appropriate use of antibiotics + **regular monthly IVIG**

NOTE: The only 2 B-cell defects for which stem cell transplantation is recommended are CD40 ligand defect (extremely rare; one of the known mutations on the X-chromosome for hyper IGM syndrome) and X-linked lymphoproliferative disease.

Common variable immunodeficiency

Common Variable Immunodeficiency (CVID) is hypogammaglobulinemia with phenotypically normal B-cells; **blood B-lymphocytes do not differentiate into IG-producing cells**

- **Genetics:** majority have no identified molecular diagnosis, so are sporadic; may have a common genetic basis with selective IgA deficiency (occurs in families together and some later with IgA may develop CVID)
- **Clinical findings:** boy or girl (**equal sex distribution**) with **later onset infections,** less severe; clinically similar to XLA, but rare echovirus meningoencephalitis
- **Diagnosis:** clinical presentation + serum IG and antibody deficiencies as profound or less than in XLA; **normal sized lymphoid tissue; later autoimmune disease and malignancy (lymphoma)**
- **Treatment:** need to be **screened for anti-IgA antibodies** (as in selective IgA deficiency)→ if present, therapy consists of the one IG preparation available that contains no IgA.

Selective IgA deficiency

Selective IgA deficiency is the **most common immunodeficiency**. It is caused by the absence or near absence of serum and secretory IgA with phenotypically normal B-cells

- **Genetics:** basic defect is unknown; boys and girls and **familial pattern** suggests autosomal dominant with variable expression; **also seen in families with CVID** (as above); both may be triggered by environmental factors
- **Clinical findings:** same bacteria as others with most infections in **respiratory, GI and urogenital** tracts; giardiasis is common

- **Diagnosis: very low-to-absent serum IgA with other IGs normal**; as with CVID, incidence of autoantibodies, autoimmune disease and malignancy increased; **serum antibodies to IgA can cause severe anaphylactic reactions if any blood product with IgA is administered (NOT a transfusion reaction)**

- **Treatment: IVIG is not indicated** (95–99% is IgG) because if usual IVIG (containing IgA) product is given, patients are at risk for severe reaction. Additionally, because it is specifically an IgA deficiency, the IVIG product with the IgA removed cannot be used. Treat the infections (generally milder).

Defects of Cellular Immunity (T-cell defects)

DiGeorge syndrome (thymic hypoplasia)

DiGeorge syndrome is thymic and parathyroid hypoplasia to aplasia from **dysmorphogenesis of the 3rd and 4th pharyngeal pouches**. Other structures are also involved: great vessel anomalies (right-sided aortic arch, interrupted aortic arch), esophageal atresia, bifid uvula, congenital heart disease (conotruncal malformations, septal defects), facial dysmorphism (short philtrum, thin upper lip, hypertelorism, mandibular hypoplasia, low-set, often notched ears), and cleft palate.

- **Genetics: microdeletions of 22q11.2** (DiGeorge syndrome chromosomal region, DGCR); 22q deletions also seen in velocardiolfacial syndrome and conotruncal anomaly face syndrome (**CATCH 22 syndromes:** Cardiac, Abnormal facies, Thymic hypoplasia, Cleft palate, Hypocalcemia); partial DiGeorge is more common, with variable thymic and parathyroid hypoplasia. About 1/3 with complete DiGeorge have the **CHARGE association**. Must confirm diagnosis for complete form by molecular genetics (fatal without definitive treatment).

- **Clinical findings:** from almost no infections with normal growth to **severe opportunistic infections and graft-versus-host disease. In most, initial presentation is neonatal hypocalcemic seizures.**

- **Diagnosis:** most with only moderately low absolute lymphocyte counts with variably decreased CD3 T-lymphocytes per the degree of thymic hypoplasia and variable response to mitogen stimulation. **Must get a T-cell count on all infants born with primary hypoparathyroidism, CHARGE, truncus arteriosus and interrupted aortic arch**

- **Treatment:** complete form correctable with either culture unrelated thymic tissue transplants or bone marrow or peripheral blood transplantation from HLA-identical sibling

Combined Antibody and Cellular Immunodeficiencies

Severe combined immunodeficiency

Severe Combined Immunodeficiency (SCID) is the absence of all **adaptive immune function**, and in some, **natural killer cells** due to diverse mutations. It is the most severe immunodeficiency known.

- **Genetics:** mutations of any one of 13 genes encoding the components of immune system critical for lymphoid cell development; result in very small thymuses which

Note

The rest of the isolated T-cell defects are extremely rare, known only to immunologists. They are not seen on the exam.

fail to descend from the neck and a lack of normal components + splenic depletion of lymphocytes and absent (or very undeveloped) remaining lymphatic tissue. X-linked SCID is the most common form in the United States.

- **Clinical findings: first 1-3 months of life with recurrent/persistent diarrhea and opportunistic infections that may lead to death; also at risk for graft-versus-host disease from maternal immunocompetent T-cells that crossed the placenta in utero**
  - **If patient continues to live without treatment, typical B-cell related infections will develop**

- **Diagnosis:** all patients have lymphopenia from birth, low-to-absent T-cells and absence of lymphocyte proliferative response to mitogens low-to-absent serum IGs and no antibodies after immunizations. The X-linked form has a low percentage of T and NK cells; autosomal recessive form more common in Europe (mutated forms in 12 genes). ADA deficiency affects primarily T-cell function (most severe lymphopenia from birth; second most common form; deletions of chromosome 20).

- **Treatment: stem cell transplantation** (HLA-identical or T-cell depleted half-matched parental); without it, most patients will die in first year but if diagnosed in first 3-4 months and treated, 94% will survive. The ADA form and X-linked have been treated with somatic gene therapy.

Combined immunodeficiency

Combined immunodeficiency is the **presence of low but not absent T-cell function and low but not absent antibodies;** patients survive longer but have failure-to-thrive and still die relatively early in life which are:

Wiskott-Aldrich syndrome

Wiskott-Aldrich Syndrome is an impaired humoral immune response and highly variable concentrations of the IGs with moderately reduced T-cells and variable mitogen responses.

- **Genetics: X-linked recessive** (Xp11.22-11.23); encodes a cytoplasmic protein restricted in expression to hematopoietic cell lines (WASP = Wiskott-Aldrich Syndrome Protein)

- **Clinical findings:** (1) thrombocytopenia presenting in neonatal period or early infancy most commonly with prolonged circumcision bleeding or bloody diarrhea, (2) atopic dermatitis, and (3) recurrent infections in first year of life (early encapsulated bacteria causing otitis, pneumonia, meningitis and sepsis, then later opportunistic infections)

- **Diagnosis:** clinical and molecular genetics; most common IG pattern is low IgM, high IgA and IgE and normal to slightly low IgG and variably reduced T-cells.

- **Treatment:** rare survival beyond adolescence (bleeding, infections and EBV-associated malignancies and autoimmune complications) without a **bone marrow transplant**

Ataxia-telangiectasia

Ataxia-telangiectasia is a moderately depressed response to T and B-cell mitogens, moderately reduced CD3 and CD4 T-cells with normal or increased percentages of CD8, T-helper cell and intrinsic B-cell defects, and hypoplastic thymus.

- **Genetics:** AT mutation (ATM) at 11.22-23
- **Clinical findings:** (1) ataxia evident with onset of walking and progresses until age 10-12 years when confined to a wheelchair (2) oculocutaneous telangiectasias develop at 3-6 years of age and (3) recurrent sinopulmonary infections most with common viruses and occasional fatal varicella; lymphoreticular malignancies and adenocarcinomas develop later; unaffected relatives also have increased incidence of malignancies
- **Treatment:** supportive care

Disorders of Phagocytic Function

Leukocyte adhesion deficiency

Leukocyte adhesion deficiency is a rare disorder of leukocyte function causing recurrent bacterial and fungal infections and **decreased inflammatory responses in the presence of neutrophilia (increased counts).**

- **Genetics:** autosomal recessive with 3 types; affects neutrophil adhesion; mutation of 21q22.3 (results in decreased expression of β_2-integrin to the endothelial surface, exiting of neutrophils from the circulation and adhesion to microorganisms (which promotes phagocytosis and activation of NAPH oxidase)
- **Clinical findings:** infant with recurrent, **low-grade bacterial infections of the skin, large chronic oral ulcers with polymicrobes and severe gingivitis; respiratory tract and genital mucosa; delayed separation of the umbilical cord with omphalitis; typical signs of inflammation may be absent and there is no pus formation; most common organisms are *S. aureus,* gram-negatives and *Candida and Aspergillus***
- **Diagnosis: paucity of neutrophils in affected tissue but circulating neutrophil count is significantly elevated;** assessment of neutrophil and monocyte adherence, aggregation, chemotaxis and phagocytosis are all abnormal diagnosis confirmed with flow cytometry showing low CD15 on neutrophils
- **Treatment:** early allogenic stem-cell transplantation for severe forms otherwise supportive care

Chronic granulomatous disease

Chronic granulomatous disease (CGD) is when neutrophils and monocytes phagocytize but cannot kill **catalase-positive microorganisms as a result of a defect in production of oxidative metabolites.**

- **Genetics/pathogenesis:** one **X-lined** and 3 autosomal recessive genes; most are **males** with X-linked inheritance; neutrophils do not produce **hydrogen peroxide, which usually acts as a substrate for myeloperoxidase** needed to oxidize halide to hypochlorous acid and chloramines that kill microbes; if organism is **catalase**

positive, the organism's hydrogen peroxide is metabolized and the organism survives, **while catalase-negative organisms survive**

- **Clinical findings:** variable age on onset and severity; **recurrent abscesses** (skin, lymph nodes, liver), pneumonia, osteomyelitis; most common pathogens are *S aureus* and then *S marcesens, B cepacia,* **Aspergillus and C. albicans,** *Nocardia and Salmonella;* granuloma formation (due to abnormal accumulation of ingested material) and inflammatory processes are the hallmark (pyloric outlet obstruction, bladder or ureteral obstruction, rectal fistulae or granulomatous colitis

- **Diagnosis:** flow cytometry using **dihydrorhodamine 123 (DHR) to measure oxidant production through increased fluorescence when oxidized by hydrogen peroxide (has taken the place of the NBT);** identifying specific genetic subgroup is useful for genetic counseling and prenatal diagnosis

- **Treatment:** only cure is stem cell transplant; otherwise supportive care including interferon to reduce serious infections

OTHER IMMUNE DEFICIENCIES

Chediak-Higashi Syndrome

- Autosomal recessive
- Abnormal secretory/storage granules lead to large and irregular seen in neutrophils
- Oculocutaneous albinism from birth, prolonged bleeding time, peripheral neuropathy, recurrent infections
- Bone marrow transplant or death from infection or lymphoproliferative-like disorder

Complement Deficiencies (rare)

- Total hemolytic complement screens for most disease of the system; it depends on all 11 components of the classical system; alternative pathway activity (D and B factors) and properdin can be diagnosed with a different assay (AP_{50})

- All components are autosomal recessive or co-dominant, except for properdin deficiency which is X-linked recessive

- Decrease in both C3 and C4 suggests activation of the alternative pathway; this is most useful in distinguishing nephritis secondary to immune complex deposition from that due to nephritic factor

- Defect in complement function: recurrent angioedema, autoimmune disease, chronic nephritis, HUS, recurrent pyogenic infections, disseminated meningococcal or gonococcal infections or a second episode of bacteremia at any age; high incidence of pneumococcal and meningococcal infections

- The only significant one (in terms of numbers of people) is ineffective synthesis of active C1 inhibitor which produces hereditary angioedema.

Graft-Versus-Host Disease (GVHD)

- Major cause of morbidity and mortality after allogenic stem cell transplantation
- Caused by engraftment of immunocompetent donor lymphocytes in an immuno-compromised host that shows histocompatibility differences with the donor lead to donor T-cell activation against recipient major or minor MHC antigens
- Acute GVHD: 2-5 weeks post-transplant; erythematous maculopapular rash, persistent anorexia, vomiting and/or diarrhea and abnormal liver enzymes and LFTs; primary prevention is with post-transplant immunosuppressive drugs and corticosteroids
- Chronic GVHD: develops or persists >3 months after transplant; major cause of non-relapse morbidity and mortality in long-term transplant survivors
    - Disorder of immune regulation: autoantibody production, increased collagen deposition and fibrosis and signs and symptoms of autoimmune disease

Disorders of the Eye 11

Learning Objectives

❏ Answer questions about congenital and acquired abnormalities of the eye structures

❏ Recognize and describe treatment approaches to periorbital versus orbital cellulitis

ABNORMALITIES OF THE EYE STRUCTURES

Pupils and iris

- **Coloboma of iris**
  - Often autosomal dominant
  - Defect of lid, iris, lens, retina, or choroid
  - Always inferior—**keyhole appearance of iris; in lid, manifests as cleft**
  - **Possible CHARGE association**
- **Leucokoria—white reflex**
  - **Retinoblastoma**
  - **Cataract**
  - Retinopathy of prematurity
  - Retinal detachment
  - Larval granulomatosis

Lens

- Cataracts—lens opacities; the most important congenital etiologies:
  - Prematurity (many disappear in a few weeks)
  - Inherited—most autosomal dominant
  - Congenital infection—TORCH (especially **rubella**); also, measles, polio, influenza, varicella, vaccinia
  - **Galactosemia**
  - Chromosomal (trisomies, deletions and duplications, XO)
  - Drugs, toxins, and trauma (**steroids**, contusions, penetrations)
- Ectopia lentis—instability or displacement of lens; edge of displaced lens may be visible in pupillary aperture
  - Differential:
    - **Trauma—most common**
    - Uveitis, congenital glaucoma, cataract, aniridia, tumor

○ Systemic causes: **Marfan syndrome** (most with superior and temporal; bilateral), **homocystinuria** (inferior and nasal), **Ehlers-Danlos**

Ocular muscles

- **Strabismus**
  - Definition—Misalignment of the eyes from abnormal innervation of muscles
  - Diagnosis—**Hirschberg corneal light reflex**—most rapid and easily performed; **light reflex should be symmetric and slightly nasal to center of each pupil**
  - Patch the good eye to eliminate amblyopia, then eye muscle surgery
- Pseudostrabismus
  - Epicanthal folds and broad nasal bridge
  - Caused by unique facial characteristics of infant
  - Transient pseudostrabismus; common up to age 4 months

Conjunctiva

A 12-hour-old newborn is noted to have bilateral conjunctival injection, tearing, and some swelling of the left eyelid. Physical examination is otherwise normal.

- **Ophthalmia neonatorum**
  - Redness, chemosis, edema of eyelids, purulent discharge
  - Causes:
    ○ Chemical conjunctivitis **most common in first 24 hours of life**
    ○ From silver nitrate and erythromycin
    ○ *N. gonorrhea*—**2–5-day incubation**; may be delayed >5 days due to suppression from prophylactic eye treatment; mild inflammatory and serosanguineous discharge, then thick and purulent; complications are corneal **ulceration**, perforation, iridocyclitis
    ○ *C. trachomatis*—**5–14-day incubation; most common;** mild inflammation to severe swelling with purulent discharge; mainly **tarsal conjunctivae**; cornea rarely affected
  - **Diagnosis—Gram stain, culture, PCR (polymerase chain reaction) for chlamydia**
  - Treatment:
    ○ *N. gonorrhea*: ceftriaxone × 1 dose IM + saline irrigation until clear
    ○ Chlamydia: erythromycin PO × 2 weeks + saline irrigation until clear (may prevent subsequent pneumonia)
- **The red eye**
  - Bacterial conjunctivitis
    ○ General conjunctival hyperemia, edema, **mucopurulent exudate** (crusting of lids together), and eye discomfort
    ○ Unilateral or bilateral
    ○ *S. pneumonia, H. influenza* (non-typable), *S. aureus*, other strep
    ○ Treatment—warm compresses and **topical antibiotics**

Note

Chemical: first day

Gonorrhea: first week

Chlamydia: second week (most common)

Note

Congenital **nasolacrimal duct obstruction** (dacryostenosis)

- Failure of canalization of duct as it enters the nose
- Excessive tears, **mucoid material** that is produced in the lacrimal sac, erythema
- Treatment— **nasolacrimal massage** 2–3×/day and warm water cleansing
- Most resolve <1 year of age

Note

Topical erythromycin *does not* prevent chlamydia conjunctivitis.

- Viral conjunctivitis
  - **Watery discharge, bilateral, usually with URI**
  - Adenovirus, enterovirus
  - Epidemic keratoconjunctivitis = adenovirus type 8
  - Good hand-washing

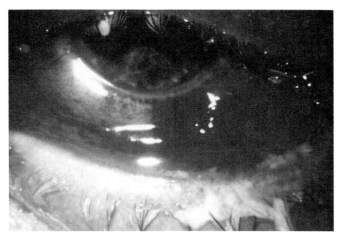

phil.cdc.gov.

Figure 11-1. Purulent, Bacterial Conjunctivitis Secondary to Gonococcal Infection of the Eye

- Allergic
- Chemical
  - Household **cleaning substances**, sprays, smoke, smog
  - Extensive tissue damage, loss of sight
- Keratitis—**corneal** involvement
  - **H. simplex, adenovirus**, *S. pneumoniae*, *S. aureus*, pseudomonas, chemicals
- Foreign bodies → corneal abrasion (pain, photophobia)
- Anterior uveitis = iridocyclitis (from ciliary body to iris)
- Periorbital versus orbital cellulitis (*see below*)
- Dacryocystitis (*S. aureus, H. influenza, S. pneumoniae*), dacroadenitis (*S. aureus*, streptococci, CMV [cytomegalovirus], measles, EBV [Epstein-Barr virus], trauma)
- Treatment—underlying cause and topical steroids

Retina and vitreous

- Retinopathy of prematurity (ROP)
  - **Prematurity, hyperoxia, and general illness**
  - From mild to severe progressive **vasoproliferative scarring** and blinding retinal detachment
  - Treatment—**cryosurgery or laser photocoagulation**

- Retinoblastoma
  - **Most common primary malignant intraocular tumor**
    - Recessive-suppressive gene—13q14 → family members need to be screened
  - Average age of diagnosis = 15 months for bilateral and 25 months for unilateral
    - **Rarely discovered at birth**
  - Initial sign in most = **leucokoria**
    - Appears as **white mass**
    - Second most common—**strabismus**
  - Diagnosis—**CT scan** to confirm; **no biopsy** (spreads easily)
  - Need to **consider enucleation**—radiation, chemotherapy, laser therapy, cryotherapy
  - Prognosis poor if extends into orbit or optic nerve

EYE INJURIES

Corneal abrasions

- Symptoms—**pain, tearing**, photophobia, decreased vision
- Diagnosis—first anesthetize eye, then **fluorescein and blue-filtered light (Wood's lamp)**
- Treatment—**pain relief and topical antibiotics**

Foreign body

- Topical anesthetic and irrigation to remove
- If embedded, send to ophthalmologist

PERIORBITAL VERSUS ORBITAL CELLULITIS

Periorbital cellulitis

- Inflammation of **lids and periorbital tissue** without signs of true orbital involvement; insidious onset; low-grade fever; no toxicity
- Causes—**trauma, infected wound**, abscess of lid, **sinusitis, bacteremia** (*H. influenza* **nontypable**, *S. pneumoniae, S. aureus*)
- May be first sign of sinusitis that may progress to orbital cellulitis
  - Physical exam: inflammation with intact eye movements; normal vision; no proptosis
- Diagnosis—clinical (blood culture unlikely to be positive)
- Treatment—**oral or IV (depending on severity) antibiotics (cover for *S. aureus* and gram positive resistant strains)**

Orbital cellulitis

A 7-year-old boy presents with swelling around the eye 2 days after suffering an insect bite to the eyelid. There is edema, erythema, and proptosis of the eye. Marked limitation of eye movements are noted. He has a low-grade fever.

- Infection of orbital tissue including subperiosteal and retrobulbar abscesses
- Physical examination
  - Ophthalmoplegia (**eyeball does not move**)
  - Chemosis
  - Inflammation
  - Proptosis
- Toxicity, fever, leukocytosis, acute onset
- Causes: **paranasal sinusitis, direct infection from wound, bacteremia**
- Organisms **nontypable** *H. influenza, S. aureus*, **beta hemolytic strep**, *S. pneumoniae*, anaerobes
- Diagnosis—CT scan with contrast of orbits and surrounding area (**best initial test**)
- Treatment—**Intravenous antibiotics (again, cover for** *S. aureus***) and may require sinus and/or orbital drainage** (will give you culture and sensitivities) if no improvement

Learning Objectives

❑ Describe diagnosis and treatment of disorders of the ears, nose, and throat in childhood

EARS

External Ear

Otitis externa (swimmer's ear)

- Normal flora of external canal includes *Pseudomonas aeruginosa* (**most common cause**), *S. aureus* (**second most common cause**), coagulase-negative *Staphylococcus*, diphtheroids, *Micrococcus* spp., and viridans streptococci
- Causes—excessive wetness, dryness, skin pathology, or trauma
- Symptoms—**significant pain** (especially with **manipulation of outer ear**), conductive hearing loss
- Findings—edema, erythema, and **thick otorrhea,** preauricular nodes
- Malignant external otitis is invasive to temporal bone and skull base—with facial paralysis, vertigo, other cranial nerve abnormalities
  - **Requires immediate culture, intravenous antibiotics, and imaging (CT scan) → may need surgery**
- Treatment   **topical otic preparations ± corticosteroids**
- Prevention—**ear plugs, thorough drying of canal, and 2% acetic acid after getting wet**

Middle Ear

Otitis media (OM)

A 4-year-old child is seen in the office with a 3-day history of fever and cold symptoms, and now complains of right ear pain. Physical examination is remarkable for a bulging tympanic membrane with loss of light reflex and landmarks.

- Acute, suppurative otitis media; accompanied by a variable degree of hearing loss (20–30 dB)

- Etiology
  - Bacterial in up to 75%
    - ○ **S. pneumoniae** (40%)
    - ○ **Nontypeable H. influenzae** (25–30%)
    - ○ **Moraxella catarrhalis** (10–15%)
  - Other 5%—Group A strep, *S. aureus*, gram negatives (neonates and hospitalized very young infants), respiratory viruses (rhinovirus, RSV most often)

Some Correlated Factors of Otitis Media

- Age: most in first 2 years
- Sex: boys > girls
- Race: more in Native Americans, Inuit
- SES: more with poverty
- Genetic: heritable component
- Breast milk versus formula: protective effect of breast milk
- Tobacco smoke: positive correlation
- Exposure to other children: positive correlation
- Season: cold weather
- Congenital anomalies: more with palatal clefts, other craniofacial anomalies, and Down syndrome

---

- Pathogenesis
  - Interruption of normal eustachian tube function (ventilation) by obstruction → inflammatory response → middle ear effusion → infection; most with URI
  - Shorter and more horizontal orientation of tube in infants and young children allows for reflux from pharynx (and in certain ethnic groups and syndromes)
- Clinical findings—highly variable
  - Symptoms—ear pain, fever, purulent otorrhea (ruptured tympanic membrane), irritability, or no symptoms
  - Pneumatic otoscopy—fullness/bulging or extreme retraction, intense erythema (otherwise erythema may be from crying, fever, sneezing; erythema alone is insufficient unless intense), some degree of opacity (underlying effusion)
  - Mobility is the most sensitive and specific factor to determine presence of a middle ear effusion (pneumatic otoscopy)
- Diagnosis—must have:
  - Acute onset
  - Tympanic membrane inflammation
  - Middle ear effusion
- Treatment—It is advisable to use routine antimicrobial treatment especially for age <2 years or those systemically ill, with severe infection, or with a history of recurrent acute otitis media.

- Pain relief is essential: acetaminophen, NSAIDs (except acetylsalicylic acid because of risk of Reye syndrome)
- **First-line drug of choice = amoxicillin (high dose)**
- **Alternate first-line drug or history of penicillin allergy = azithromycin**
- In some patients age >2 years who do not have high fevers or severe pain, the physician may just observe and reevaluate in 2-3 days. If no improvement or if any worsening, antibiotics should then be started.
- Duration—10 days; shorter if mild, older child
- Follow up—within days for young infants, continued pain or severe; otherwise 2 weeks (sustained improvement seen in TM)
- **Second-line drugs—if continued pain after 2–3 days**
  - **Amoxicillin — clavulinic acid** (effective against β-lactamase producing strains)
  - Cefuroxime axetil (unpalatable, low acceptance)
  - **IM ceftriaxone (may need repeat 1–2×; for severe infection if oral not possible), if patient is not taking/tolerating oral medications**
  - Also maybe cefdinir (very palatable, shorter duration)
  - If **clinical response to good second-line drug is unsatisfactory,** perform myringotomy or tympanoscentesis

Otitis media with effusion (OME)

- Generally after repeated infections with insufficient time for effusion to resolve
- **Fullness is absent or slight or TM retracted; no or very little erythema**
- Treatment
  - Monthly evaluation
  - Assess hearing if effusion >3 months; most resolve without problems
  - **Recent studies suggest that in otherwise healthy children an effusion up to 9 months in both ears during first 3 years of life poses no developmental risks at 3–4 years of life.**
  - **Routine antibiotic prophylaxis is *not* recommended.**
  - **Tympanostomy tubes**
    - **Suggested for children with bilateral OME and impaired hearing for >3 months; prolonged unilateral or bilateral OME with symptoms (school or behavioral problems, vestibular, ear discomfort); or prolonged OME in cases of risk for developmental difficulties (Down syndrome, craniofacial disorders, developmental disorders).**
    - Likelihood that middle ear ventilation will be sustained for at least as long as tubes remain in (average 12 months)
- Complications
  - Acute mastoiditis—**displacement of pinna** inferiorly and anteriorly and inflammation of posterior auricular area; pain on percussion of mastoid process
    - Diagnosis—When suspected or diagnosed clinically, perform CT scan of temporal bone.
    - Treatment—**myringotomy and IV antibiotics** (*S. pneumoniae*, nontypable *H. influenzae, P. aeroginosa*); if bone destruction, intravenous antibiotics and mastoidectomy

Note

Abnormal Exam Findings

Purulent otorrhea–sign of otitis externa, otitis media with perforation and/or drainage from middle ear through tympanostomy tube

Bulging TM–increased middle ear pressure with pus or effusion in middle ear

TM retraction–negative middle ear pressure (more rapid diffusion of air from middle ear cavity than its replacement via the eustachian tube)

Other findings for an effusion–bubbles, air-fluid level seen behind TM

- **Acquired cholesteatoma** = cyst-like growth within middle ear or temporal bone; lined by keratinized, stratified squamous epithelium
  - Most with long-standing chronic otitis media
  - **Progressively expands**—bony resorption and intracranially; life-threatening
  - **Discrete, white opacity of eardrum** through a defect in TM or persistent malodorous ear discharge
  - **CT scan** to define presence and extent
  - Treatment—**tympanomastoid surgery**

NOSE AND THROAT

Nose

Choanal atresia

A newborn is noted to be cyanotic in the wellborn nursery. On stimulation, he cries and becomes pink again. The nurse has difficulty passing a catheter through the nose.

- Unilateral or bilateral bony (most) or membranous septum between nose and pharynx
  - Half have other anomalies (**CHARGE** association)
  - Unilateral—asymptomatic for long time until first URI, then persistent nasal discharge with obstruction
  - Bilateral—**typical pattern of cyanosis while trying to breathe through nose, then becoming pink with crying**; if can breathe through mouth, will have problems while feeding
- Diagnosis
  - Inability to pass catheter 3–4 cm into nasopharynx
  - Fiberoptic rhinoscopy
  - Best way to delineate anatomy is CT scan
- Treatment
  - Establish oral airway, possible intubation
  - Transnasal repair with stent(s)

Foreign body
- Any small object
- Clinical—unilateral **purulent, malodorous bloody discharge**
- Diagnosis—may be seen with nasal speculum or otoscope; lateral skull film if radiopaque (may have been pushed back, embedded in granulation tissue)
- Treatment—if cannot easily remove with needle-nose forceps, refer to ENT

Epistaxis

An 8-year-old child has repeated episodes of nosebleeds. Past history, family history, and physical examination are unremarkable.

- Common in childhood; decreases with puberty
- Most common area—**anterior septum** (Kiesselbach plexus), prone to exposure
- Etiology
    - **Digital trauma** (nose picking; most common)
    - **Dry air (especially winter)**
    - **Allergy**
    - **Inflammation (especially with URI)**
    - **Nasal steroid sprays**
    - Severe GERD in young infants
    - Congenital vascular anomalies
    - Clotting disorders, hypertension
- Treatment—most stop spontaneously
    - Compress nares, upright, head forward; cold compress
    - If this does not work, then **local oxymetazolone or phenylephrine**
    - If this does not work, then **anterior nasal packing**; if it appears to be coming posteriorly, need **posterior nasal packing**
    - If bleeding site identified, **cautery**
    - Use humidifier, saline drops, petrolatum for prevention

Polyps

- Benign pedunculated tumors from chronically inflamed nasal mucosa
    - Usually from ethmoid sinus external to middle meatus
- **Most common cause is cystic fibrosis—suspect in any child <12 years old with polyp; EVEN in absence of other typical symptoms**
- May also be associated with the Samter triad (polyps, aspirin sensitivity, asthma)
- Presents with **obstruction** → hyponasal speech and mouth breathing; may have profuse mucopurulent rhinorrea
- Examination—generally glistening, gray, grape-like masses
- Treatment—**intranasal steroids/systemic steroids may provide some shrinkage (helpful in CF);** remove surgically if complete obstruction, uncontrolled rhinorrhea, or nose deformity.

Sinusitis

- Acute—viral versus bacterial
- Most with URI—most viral, self-limited; up to 2% complicated by bacterial sinusitis
- Sinus development
    - Ethmoid and maxillary present at birth, but only **ethmoid is pneumatized**

- – Sphenoid present by 5 years
- – Frontal begins at 7–8 years and not completely developed until adolescence
- Etiology—*S. pneumonia*, **nontypeable** *H. influenzae, M. catarrhalis; S. aureus* **in chronic cases**
  - – May occur at **any age**
  - – Predisposed with URI, allergy, cigarette smoke exposure
  - – Chronic—immune deficiency, CF, ciliary dysfunction, abnormality of phagocytic function, GERD, cleft palate, nasal polyps, nasal foreign body
- Pathophysiology—fluid in sinuses during most URIs from nose blowing. Inflammation and edema may block sinus drainage and impair clearance of bacteria.
- Clinical features
  - – **Nonspecific complaints—nasal congestion, discharge, fever, cough**
  - – Less commonly—bad breath, decreased sense of smell, periorbital edema headache, face pain
  - – Sinus tenderness only in adolescents and adults; exam mostly shows mild erythema and swelling of nasal mucosa and discharge
- Diagnosis—**entirely historical and clinical presentation (evidence-based)**
  - – **Persistent URI symptoms without improvement for at least 10 days**
  - – **Severe respiratory symptoms with purulent discharge and temperature at least 38.9°C (102°F) for at least 3 consecutive days**
    - ○ Only accurate method to distinguish viral versus bacterial is sinus aspirate and culture, but this is NOT done routinely
    - ○ Sinus films/CT scans—show mucosal thickening, opacification, air-fluid levels, but does not distinguish viral versus bacterial
- Treatment
  - – Initial—amoxicillin (adequate for majority)
  - – Alternative—cefuroxime axetil, cefpodoxime, azithromycin
  - – Treat 7 days past improvement
  - – If still does not work—to ENT (maxillary sinus aspirate)

Note

The same organisms that are responsible for AOM are also implicated in sinusitis.

Throat

Acute pharyngitis

An 8-year-old girl complains of acute sore throat of 2 day's duration, accompanied by fever and mild abdominal pain. Physical examination reveals enlarged, erythematous tonsils with exudate and enlarged, slightly tender cervical lymph nodes.

- Viruses versus group A beta-hemolytic strep (GABHS)
- Viral—typical winter and spring; close contact
- GABHS—**uncommon <2–3 years of age**; increased incidence in childhood, then decreases in adolescence; **all year long** (but most in cold months)

- Clinical presentation
  - Strep pharyngitis
    - **Rapid onset**
    - **Severe sore throat and fever**
    - **Headache and gastrointestinal symptoms frequently**
    - **Exam—red pharynx, tonsilar enlargement with yellow, blood-tinged exudate, petechiae on palate and posterior pharynx, strawberry tongue, red swollen uvula, increased and tender anterior cervical nodes**
  - Scarlet fever—from GABHS that produce one of three streptococcal pyogenic exotoxins (SPE A, B, C); **exposure to each confers a specific immunity to that toxin, and so one can have scarlet fever up to three times**
    - Findings of pharyngitis plus **circumoral pallor**
    - **Red, finely papular erythematous rash diffusely that feels like sandpaper**
    - Pastia's lines in intertriginous areas
  - Viral—more gradual; with typical URI symptoms; erythematous pharynx, no pus
    - Pharyngoconjunctival fever (adenovirus)
    - **Coxsackie:**
      - Herpangina—small 1–2 mm vesicles and ulcers on posterior pharynx
      - Acute lymphonodular pharyngitis—small 3–6 mm yellowish-white nodules on posterior pharynx with lymphadenopathy
      - **Hand-foot-mouth disease—inflamed oropharynx with scattered vesicles on tongue, buccal mucosa, gingiva, lips, and posterior pharynx → ulcerate; also on hands and feet and buttocks; tend to be painful**
- Diagnosis of strep
  - First—**rapid strep test; if positive, do not need throat culture**
    - **But must confirm a negative rapid test with cultures if clinical suspicion is high**
- Treatment—early treatment only hastens recovery by 12–24 hours **but prevents acute rheumatic fever if treated within 9 days of illness**
  - **Penicillin**
  - **Allergy—erythromycin**
- Complications
  - Retropharyngeal and lateral pharyngeal abscess—deep nodes in neck; infection from extension of localized infection of oropharynx
    - Clinical—nonspecific—fever, irritability, decreased oral intake, **neck stiffness, torticollis, refusal to move neck, muffled voice**
    - **Examination—bulging of posterior or lateral pharyngeal wall**
    - Soft tissue neck film with head extended may show increase width
    - Definitive diagnosis—incision and drainage, **C and S—most polymicrobial (GABHS, anaerobes, *S. aureus*)**
    - **Treatment**
      - Intravenous antibiotics ± surgical drainage
      - **Third-generation cephalosporin plus ampicillin/sulbactam or clindamycin**
      - **Surgical drainage needed if respiratory distress or failure to improve**

Note

Causes of Cervical Lymphadenitis

- Infections
  - Viral/baceterial pharyngitis
  - Cat scratch disease
  - Tb/atypical mycobacteria
  - Mumps
  - Thyroglossal duct cyst
  - Branchial cleft cyst
- Cystic hygroma
- Tumors (rare)

- Peritonsillar abscess—bacterial invasion through capsule of tonsil
  - Typical presentation—adolescent with recurrent history of acute pharyngotonsillitis
  - Sore throat, fever, dysphagia, trismus
  - Examination—**asymmetric tonsillar bulge with displacement of uvula away from the affected side is diagnostic**
  - GABHS + mixed oropharyngeal anaerobes
  - Treatment
    - Antibiotics and **needle aspiration**
    - **Incision and drainage**
    - **Tonsillectomy if recurrence or complications (rupture with aspiration)**

Indications for tonsillectomy, and adenoidectomy

- Tonsillectomy
  - Rate of strep pharyngitis: ≥**7 documented** infections within past year or 5/year for 2 years or 3/year for 3 years
  - Unilateral enlarged tonsil (neoplasm most likely but rare)
- Adenoidectomy
  - Chronic nasal/sinus infection failing medical treatment
  - Recurrent/chronic OM in children with tympanostomy tubes and persistent otorrhea
  - Nasal obstruction with chronic mouth-breathing and loud snoring
- Tonsillectomy and adenoidectomy
  - ≥ 7 infections
  - Upper airway obstruction secondary to hypertrophy resulting in sleep-disordered breathing and complications

Cardiology 13

Learning Objectives

❑ Demonstrate understanding of the pediatric cardiac evaluation

❑ Categorize disorders in which left-to-right shunt, right-to-left shunt, or hypertension occurs

❑ Recognize stenotic, regurgitant, and mixed disorders

❑ Cardiac evaluation and congenital heart lesions

CARDIAC EVALUATION AND CONGENITAL HEART LESIONS

Children do not present with the typical features of congestive heart failure as seen in adults. Age is very important when assessing the child.

- Infants:
  - Feeding difficulties
  - Easily fatigued
  - Sweating while feeding
  - Rapid respirations
- Older children:
  - Shortness of breath
  - Dyspnea on exertion
- Physical examination
  - Need to refer to normal heart and respiratory rates for ages to determine tachycardia and tachypnea.
  - Height and weight should be assessed to determine proper growth.
  - Always get upper and lower extremity blood pressures and pulses.
  - Hepatosplenomegaly suggests right-sided heart failure.
  - Rales on auscultation may indicate pulmonary edema and left-sided heart failure.
  - Cyanosis and clubbing result from hypoxia.

Note

Orthopnea and nocturnal dyspnea are **rare** findings in children.

Table 13-1. Heart Murmur Gradation

Grade	Quality
1	Soft, difficult to hear
2	Easily heard
3	Louder but no thrill
4	Associated with thrill
5	Thrill; audible with edge of stethoscope
6	Thrill; audible with stethoscope just off chest

- Diagnostic tests—chest radiograph
  - Evaluate heart size, lung fields, ribs for notching, position of great vessels
  - Electrocardiogram
  - **Echocardiography—definitive diagnosis**
  - Other—MRI, cardiac catheterization, angiography, exercise testing
- Embryology—knowledge of cardiac embryology is helpful for understanding congenital cardiac lesions, their presentations, symptoms, and treatment.

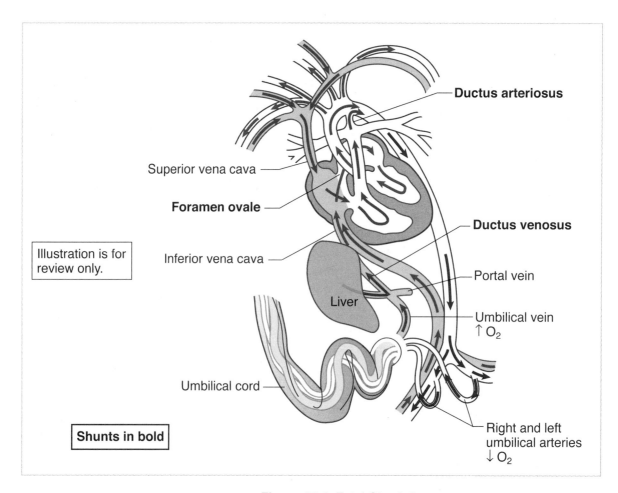

Figure 13-1. Fetal Circulation

PEDIATRIC HEART SOUNDS AND INNOCENT MURMURS

Heart Sounds

First heart sound (S1)

- Closure of mitral and tricuspid valves (MV, TV)
- High pitch, but lower pitch and greater intensity compared to S1
- Usually no discernible splitting of S1 but in completely normal child, a split S1 represents asynchronous closure of the 2 valves (20–30 msec difference); however, what sounds like a split S1 but is not represents pathology:
  - Split S1 best heard at apex or right upper sternal border may be a click (opening of stenotic valve) may be heard in aortic stenosis
  - Apical mid systolic click of mitral valve prolapse
  - At upper left sternal border, a click may be heard from pulmonic valve stenosis; compared to aortic stenosis, this changes with respiration (with inspiration, venous return is increased, thus causing the abnormal pulmonary valve to float superiorly after which the click softens or disappears)
  - Tricuspid valve abnormalities (e.g., Ebstein anomaly) may cause billowing of the leaflets and result in multiple clicks
- S1 may be inaudible at the lower left sternal border mostly due to sounds that obscure the closure of the MV and TV, e.g., in VSD, PDA, mitral or tricuspid regurgitation and severe right ventricular outflow tract obstruction. Therefore, if the **first heart sound is not heard at the lower left sternal border, there is most likely a congenital heart defect, and there will be other clinical and auscultatory findings.**

Second heart sound (S2)

- Closure of pulmonary and aortic valves (PV, AV), which close simultaneously on exhalation and a single heart sound is best heard with diaphragm at the upper left sternal border
  - **Wider splitting of S2 on inspiration is related not only to increased venous return but also to pressures in the aorta and pulmonary artery (PA) (it is significantly higher in the Ao than in the PA, so Ao valve closes first)**
- **Wider than normal splitting will occur with any lesion that allows more blood to traverse the PV compared to normal**
  - Increased splitting of S2 may be fixed with respect to respiration if there is increased volume and hence pressure in the right atrium (e.g., ASD); otherwise, it will continue to vary with respiration; may also hear fixed splitting with a right bundle branch block
- **Loud single S2**: heard with PA hypertension (increased pressure closing the PV causes early closure of the anterior semilunar valve resulting in a loud single S2)
  - In D-transposition, the AV is anterior and to the right of the PV, which overwhelms the sound from the PV, so one hears a loud single S2; in truncus arteriosus, there is only 1 valve so there is a single S2

Third heart sound (S3)

- Hear **early in diastole**; creates a gallop rhythm with S1 + S2; very low frequency and is best heard with bell of the stethoscope at cardiac apex; asking patient to lie on left side may increase intensity of S3

- **On occasion may be heard normally in children with no pathology:** in older people, it represents the presence of CHF and is caused by sudden deceleration of blood flow into LV from the LA

Fourth heart sound (S4)

- Occurs in **late diastole, just prior to S1 (presystolic) and is produced by a decrease in compliance (increased stiffness) of the LV**

- Low frequency (lower than S3) and best heard with bell of the stethoscope pressed lightly against the skin; never hear with atrial fibrillation because the contraction of the atria is ineffective

- Summation gallop rhythm (S3 + S4) may be found with improving CHF, myocarditis, or a cardiomyopathy

Innocent Murmurs

Peripheral pulmonic stenosis

- **Normal finding age 6 weeks to 1 year**

- Generated by blood flowing into the lungs due to (1) pulmonary arteries, which have limited blood flow in utero and are therefore small with significantly increased blood flow after birth (turbulence from RV blood flowing through these arteries), and (2) increasing cardiac output associated with declining [Hgb] over the first weeks of life (physiologic anemia)

- Normal infant with normal S1, then grade 1-2 systolic ejection murmur at the upper sternal border and radiating bilaterally into the axillae; then, normal splitting of S2

Still's murmur

- Commonly heard first at **age 3–5 years**

- Represents turbulence or vibrations in either ventricle; child is healthy and asymptomatic

- Precordial activity is normal, as are S1 and S2; the murmur is typically low-pitched (bell of stethoscope), musical-quality and often radiates throughout the precordium.

- Murmur is **loudest while supine (greater blood flow) and decreases sitting or standing—opposite to the finding of HOCM.** Also increases with fever or exercise (hyperdynamic states).

Venous hum

- Only diastolic murmur that is **not** pathological; **represents blood flow returning from the head and flowing from SVC into the RA**

- Described as "whooshing" sound (like holding a seashell to your ear at the ocean); is a **continuous murmur**

  - Best heard in sitting position with head in the neutral position

  - **Murmur becomes softer or disappears while in supine, with slight pressure to the right side of the neck or turning head to opposite side**

Aortic outflow murmur

- Heard **in adolescents and young adults** (especially athletes, due to lower resting heart rate and therefore larger stroke volume

- Best heard in upper right sternal border; represents blood flow in RV outflow tract (**without a click, as there is in aortic stenosis**)

- Precordial activity is normal, S1 and S2 are normal, the murmur is grade 1-2 ejection

    - Going from **supine to sitting or standing decreases the murmur** (again, opposite to HOCM)

Congenital Heart Disease

In most cases, diagnosis usually made by age 1 month. Murmurs may not be heard in early life because of increased pulmonary vascular resistance (from fetal to neonatal transition physiology).

- Etiology

    - Most are unknown

    - Associated with teratogens, such as alcohol and rubella

    - Genetic predisposition—trisomies; Marfan, Noonan, DiGeorge syndromes

- Classification

Table 13-2. Congenital Heart Disease

	Shunting			
Regurgitant	**Stenotic**	**Right → Left**	**Left → Right**	**Mixing**
MVP	Aortic stenosis	Tetralogy of Fallot	Patent ductus	Truncus
PI, AI	Pulmonic stenosis	Ebstein anomaly	Ventricular septal defect	TAPVR
MI, TI	Coarctation	Tricuspid atresia	Atrial septal defect, endocardiac cushion defect	HLH, Transposition

Definition of abbreviations: TAPVR *total anomalous pulmonary venous return;* HLH *hypoplastic left heart;* MVP *mitral valve prolapse;* PI *pulmonic insufficiency;* AI *aortic insufficiency;* MI *myocardial infarction;* TI *tricuspid insufficiency*

LEFT TO RIGHT SHUNTS

Ventricular Septal Defect (VSD)

A 3-month-old child presents with poor feeding, poor weight gain, and tachypnea. Physical examination reveals a harsh, pansystolic 3/6 murmur at the left lower sternal border, and hepatomegaly.

- **Most common** congenital heart lesion
- Most are **membranous**
- Shunt determined by **ratio of PVR to SVR**

    - **As PVR falls in first few weeks of life, shunt increases**

    - When PVR>SVR, **Eisenmenger** syndrome (must **not be allowed** to happen)

Note

Eisenmenger Syndrome

- Transformation of any untreated left-to-right shunt into a bidirectional or right-to-left shunt

- Characterized by cyanosis

- Results from high pulmonary blood flow, causing medial hypertrophy of pulmonary vessels and increased pulmonary vascular resistance

- Clinical findings
  - Asymptomatic if small defect with normal pulmonary artery pressure (most); large defect—**dyspnea, feeding difficulties, poor growth, sweating, pulmonary infection, heart failure**
  - Harsh holosystolic **murmur** over lower left sternal border ± thrill; S_2 widely split
  - With hemodynamically significant lesions, also a low-pitched diastolic rumble across the mitral valve heard best at the apex
- Diagnosis—chest-ray (large heart, pulmonary edema), ECG (LVH), echocardiogram is definitive
- Treatment
  - Small **muscular VSD more likely to close in first 1–2 years than membranous**
  - Less common for moderate to large to close → medical treatment for heart failure (**control failure and prevent pulmonary vascular disease**)
  - **Surgery in first year**; indications:
    - Failure to thrive or unable to be corrected medically
    - Infants at 6–12 months with large defects and pulmonary artery hypertension
    - More than 24 months of age with Qp:Qs >2:1 (shunt fraction)

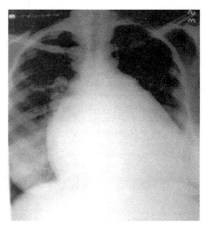

Courtesy of Tom D. Thacher, M.D.

Figure 13-2. Cardiomegaly Due to Ventricular Septal Defect

- Complications
  - Large defects lead to heart failure, failure to thrive
  - Endocarditis
  - Pulmonary hypertension

Atrial Septal Defect (ASD)

- Ostium secundum defect **most common** (in region of fossa ovalis)
- Clinical
  - **Few symptoms early in life** because of structure of low-flow, left-to-right shunt
  - In older children, often with large defects; varying degrees of exercise intolerance
  - With hemodynamically significant lesions, also a low-pitched diastolic rumble across the tricuspid valve heard best at the lower sternum

- Physical examination
  - **Wide fixed splitting of S$_2$**
  - Systolic ejection murmur along left mid to upper sternal border (from increased pulmonary flow)
- Diagnosis
  - Chest x-ray—varying heart enlargement (right ventricular and right atrial); increased pulmonary vessel markings, edema
  - ECG—**right-axis deviation and RVH**
  - Echocardiogram definitive
- Treatment
  - Most in term infants close spontaneously; **symptoms often do not appear until third decade**
  - **Surgery or transcatheter device closure for all symptomatic patients or 2:1 shunt**
- Complications
  - Dysrhythmia
  - Low-flow lesion; does not require endocarditis prophylaxis

Endocardial Cushion Defect

- Pathophysiology
  - When both ASDs and VSDs occur, which are contiguous, and the atrioventricular valves are abnormal
  - Left-to-right shunt at both atrial and ventricular levels; some right-to-left shunting with desaturation (**mild, intermittent cyanosis)**
  - Atrioventricular valve insufficiency → increase volume load on one or both ventricles; **early heart failure, infections, minimal cyanosis, hepatomegaly, and failure to thrive**
- Physical examination
  - Heart failure early in infancy (hepatomegaly, failure to thrive)
  - Eisenmenger physiology occurs earlier
  - Moderate-to-severe increase in heart size with hyperdynamic precordium (**precordial bulge and lift)**
  - **Widely fixed split S$_2$** (like an isolated ASD)
  - **Pulmonary systolic ejection murmur, low-pitched diastolic rumble at left sternal border and apex;** may also have mitral insufficiency (apical harsh holosystolic murmur radiating to left axilla)
- Diagnostic tests
  - Chest x-ray—significant cardiomegaly, increased pulmonary artery and pulmonary blood flow and edema
  - ECG—signs of biventricular hypertrophy, right atrial enlargement, superior QRS axis
  - Echocardiogram (gold standard)
- Treatment—surgery more difficult with heart failure and pulmonary hypertension (increased pulmonary artery pressure by 6–12 months of age); **must be performed in infancy**
- Complications
  - Without surgery—death from heart failure
  - With surgery—arrhythmias, congenital heart block

Note

Patients with trisomy 21 are at a higher risk for endocardial cushion defects.

Note

If a PDA persists beyond the first week of life, it is unlikely to close spontaneously.

Patent Ductus Arteriosus (PDA)

- Results when the ductus arteriosus fails to close; this leads to blood flow from the aorta to the pulmonary artery
- Risk factors
  - **More common in girls** by 2:1
  - Associated with **maternal rubella infection**
  - Common in **premature infants** (developmental, not heart disease)
- Presentation
  - If small—possibly no symptoms
  - If large—heart failure, a wide pulse pressure, bounding arterial pulses, characteristic sound of "machinery," decreased blood pressure (primarily diastolic)
- Diagnostic tests
  - Chest x-ray—increased pulmonary artery with increased pulmonary markings and edema; moderate-to-large heart size
  - ECG—left ventricular hypertrophy
  - Echocardiogram—increased left atrium to aortic root; ductal flow, especially in diastole
- Treatment
  - May close spontaneously
  - Indomethacin (preterm infants)
  - Surgical closure
- Complications
  - Congestive heart failure
  - Infective endocarditis

STENOTIC LESIONS

Pulmonic Stenosis

Note

Pulmonic stenosis as a result of valve dysplasia is the common defect in **Noonan syndrome** (12a24.1; autosomal dominant; boys and girls with Turner phenotype).

Pulmonic stenosis (either valve or branched artery) is common in **Alagille syndrome** (arteriohepatic dysplasia).

- Pathophysiology
  - Deformed cusps → opens incompletely during systole; obstruction to right ventricular outflow → increased systemic pressure and wall stress → **right ventricular hypertrophy (depends on severity of pulmonary stenosis)**
  - **Arterial saturation normal unless ASD or VSD is present with R → L shunt**
  - Neonate with severe pulmonary stenosis = critical pulmonary stenosis = R → L shunt via foramen ovale
- Physical examination
  - Heart failure only in severe cases, most in first month of life
  - Mild cases—normal life, usually no progression
  - **Moderate to severe**—increasing gradient with growth: **signs of right ventricular failure** (hepatomegaly, peripheral edema, exercise intolerance)
  - **Pulmonary ejection click** after S_1 in left upper sternal border and normal S_2 (in mild); relatively **short, low-to-medium–pitched SEM** over pulmonic area radiating to both lung fields

- Diagnosis
  - ECG—**right ventricular hypertrophy in moderate to severe**; tall, spiked P-waves; right atrial enlargement (RAE)
  - Chest x-ray—**poststenotic dilatation of pulmonary artery;** normal-to-increased heart size (right ventricle) and **decreasing pulmonary vascularity**
  - Echocardiogram (gold standard)
- Complications
  - Heart failure
  - Endocarditis (lower risk)
  - Secondary subvalvular muscular and fibrous hypertrophy
- Treatment
  - Moderate to severe—**balloon valvuloplasty** initially; may need surgery
  - Neonate with **critical pulmonary stenosis—emergent surgery**

Aortic Stenosis

- Most are **bicuspid aortic valve**—usually asymptomatic in children
- Supravalvular stenosis (least common form)—sporadic, familial, or with Williams syndrome (mental retardation, elfin facies, heart disease, idiopathic hypercalcemia; deletion of elastin gene 7q11.23)
- Clinical presentation—**symptoms depend on severity of obstruction**
  - If severe early in infancy = **critical aortic stenosis** = left ventricular failure and decreased cardiac output
  - **If significant decrease in cardiac output—intensity of murmur at right upper sternal border may be minimal**
  - Mild to moderate—usually asymptomatic with normal growth and development
    - Often discovered with murmur on routine physical examination
    - Rare—older children present with syncope, fatigue, angina, dizziness
  - **With increasing severity—decreased pulses, increased heart size, left ventricular apical thrust**
  - **Early systolic ejection click at apex of left sternal border (does not vary with respiration)**
    - Severe—no click and decreased S1 (decreased left ventricular compliance), decreased S_2 (aortic component), and maybe an S_4
    - **SEM upper-right second intercostal space; the louder (harsher) and longer the murmur, the greater the degree of obstruction; radiates to neck and left midsternal border; positive thrill in suprasternal notch**
- Diagnosis
  - ECG—**left ventricular hypertrophy** and strain
  - Chest x-ray—**prominent ascending aorta**; may have valve calcification (older children and adults); if severe → increased heart size (left ventricular hypertrophy)
  - **Echocardiogram (gold standard)**
- Treatment
  - Balloon valvuloplasty
  - Surgery on valves
  - Valve replacement

Note

Coarctation of the aorta has a high association with Turner syndrome (70% with bicuspid aortic valve).

Note

Coarctation should be suspected in an asymptomatic child with hypertension.

Coarctation of the Aorta

- Definition—narrowing at any point from transverse arch to iliac bifurcation; 90% just below origin of left subclavian artery at origin of ductus arteriosus (juxtaductal coarctation)

Adult versus childhood

- **Discrete juxtaductal coarctation (adult type)**
  - Ascending aortic blood flows normally through narrowed segment to reach descending aorta, but there is left ventricular hypertrophy and hypertension
  - If mild, not recognized until later in childhood
  - Increased blood pressure in vessels proximal to coarctation and decreased blood pressure and pulses below constriction
    - ○ Femoral and other lower pulses weak or absent; bounding in arms and carotids; also **delay in femoral pulse** compared to radial (femoral normally occurs slightly before radial)
    - ○ Normally, leg systolic pressure is 10–20 mm Hg higher than in arms; in coarctation, leg systolic pressure is decreased (>5%)
    - ○ If pressure is greater in right arm than left arm, suggests coarctation involving left subclavian artery
    - ○ Short systolic murmur along left sternal border at third-to-fourth intercostal space → left scapula and neck
  - Hypertension due not only to mechanical but also to neurohormonal reasons
  - Over time, patient develops an extensive collateral circulation (systolic or continuous murmurs over left and right sides of chest with thrills), **rib notching** (dilated intercostal arteries)
- **Tubular hypoplasia (preductal, infantile type)**
  - Severe narrowing starting at one of the head or neck vessels and extending to the ductus
  - Right ventricular blood flows across the PDA to supply the descending aorta so the perfusion of the lower part of the body is dependent upon right ventricular output
  - Seen as differential cyanosis—**upper body is pink, lower is cyanotic**; prominent heart failure as ductus closes (if completely atretic = interrupted aortic arch)
  - Presents with lower body hypoperfusion, acidosis, and severe heart failure with ductal closure; large heart, systolic murmur along left sternal border
- Diagnostic tests
  - Chest x-ray—depends on age and effects of hypertension and collaterals
    - ○ Severe (infantile)—increased heart size and pulmonary congestion
    - ○ Adult—findings usually occur after first decade:
      - ▸ Increased size of subclavian artery—prominent shadow in left superior mediastinum
      - ▸ **Notching of inferior border of ribs** from passive erosion of increased collaterals in late childhood
      - ▸ Poststenotic dilatation of ascending aorta

- Diagnosis
  - ECG—left ventricular hypertrophy in older children; in neonates, biventricular hypertrophy
  - Echocardiogram (gold standard)
- Treatment
  - Neonate—PGE$_1$ infusion to maintain patent, ductus, which establishes adequate lower extremity blood flow; **surgery** after stabilization
  - **Surgery soon after diagnosis of any significant coarctation**
  - Adult—treat heart failure and hypertension, then follow with surgery
- Complications
  - Associated cerebrovascular disease
  - Systemic hypertension
  - Endocarditis
  - Aortic aneurysms

CYANOTIC LESIONS (RIGHT TO LEFT SHUNTS)

Cyanotic Lesions Associated with Decreased Pulmonary Blood Flow

Tetralogy of Fallot (TOF)

A 6-month-old infant is prone to episodes of restlessness, cyanosis, and gasping respirations. Symptoms resolve when he is placed in the knee-chest position. Physical examination reveals an underweight infant, with a harsh long systolic ejection murmur and a single second heart sound.

- Components
  - Pulmonary stenosis and infundibular stenosis (obstruction to right ventricular outflow)
  - VSD
  - Overriding aorta (overrides the VSD)
  - Right ventricular hypertrophy
- **Most common cyanotic lesion**
- Pulmonary stenosis plus hypertrophy of subpulmonic muscle (crista supraventricularis) → varying degrees of right ventricular outflow obstruction
  - Blood shunted right-to-left across the VSD with varying degrees of arterial desaturation and cyanosis
  - **If mild, patient may not be visibly cyanotic (pink tetralogy of Fallot)**
    ○ With growth and further hypertrophy of infundibulum, cyanosis may be seen later in first year of life
  - With severe obstruction, cyanosis in the immediate neonatal period (ductal dependent)

Note

Common Cyanotic Heart Disease (5 Ts)

Tetralogy of Fallot

Transposition of great vessels

Truncus arteriosis

Total anomalous pulmonary venous return

Tricuspid atresia

- If not corrected, older children are blue, have marked clubbing, and have **dyspnea on exertion (child will squat to increase systemic vascular resistance and to decrease right-to-left shunt)**

- Paroxysmal hypercyanotic attacks (tet spells)

  ○ Acute onset of hyperpnea and restlessness → increased cyanosis → gasping → syncope (increased infundibular obstruction with further right-to-left shunting

  ○ Treatment—place in lateral knee-chest position, give oxygen, inject subcutaneous morphine, give beta-blockers

- Physical examination—substernal right ventricular impulse, systolic thrill along third-to-fourth intercostal space on left sternal border, loud and harsh systolic ejection murmur (upper sternal border), may be preceded by a click; **either a single S$_2$** or soft pulmonic component

- Diagnosis

  - Chest x-ray—hypertrophied right ventricle causes the apex to be uplifted above the diaphragm → **boot-shaped heart** plus dark lung fields (decreased pulmonary blood flow)

  - ECG—right axis deviation plus right ventricular hypertrophy

  - Echocardiogram (gold standard)

- Pre-correction complications—cerebral thromboses, brain abscess, bacterial endocarditis, heart failure, but not common because of early correction

- Treatment

  - Depends on degree of obstruction

    ○ PGE$_1$ infusion—prevent ductal closure; given if cyanotic at birth

    ○ Augment pulmonary blood flow with **palliative systemic to pulmonary shunt** (modified Blalock-Taussig shunt)

    ○ Corrective surgery (electively at age 4–12 months)—remove obstructive muscle, valvulotomy, and patching of VSD

Tricuspid atresia

- Pathophysiology—**no outlet from the right atrium to the right ventricle;** entire venous (systemic) return enters the left atrium from a foramen ovale or ASD (**there must be an atrial communication**); left ventricular blood to right ventricle (atretic) via a VSD and is augmented by PDA; **therefore, pulmonary blood flow depends on presence (and size) of VSD**

- Clinical presentation

  - Will present at birth with **severe cyanosis**

  - **Increased left ventricular impulse** (contrast to most others with right ventricular impulse), holosystolic murmurs along left sternal border (most have a VSD; though right ventricle is small, it is still a conduit for pulmonary blood flow)

- Diagnosis

  - Chest x-ray—**pulmonary undercirculation**

  - ECG—**left axis deviation plus left ventricular hypertrophy** (distinguishes from most other congenital heart disease)

  - Echocardiogram (gold standard)

Note

The combination of severe cyanosis in the newborn *plus* a chest x-ray showing decreased pulmonary blood flow *plus* an ECG with left axis deviation and left ventricular hypertrophy is most likely to be **tricuspid atresia.**

- Treatment
  - **PGE_1 until aortopulmonary shunt can be performed**
  - May need an **atrial balloon septostomy (to make larger ASD)**
  - Later, staged surgical correction

Ebstein anomaly

- Development associated with periconceptional maternal **lithium** use in some cases
- **Downward displacement of abnormal tricuspid valve into right ventricle;** the right ventricle gets divided into two parts: an atrialized portion, which is thin-walled, and smaller normal ventricular myocardium
- **Right atrium is huge; tricuspid valve regurgitant**
- **Right ventricular output is decreased** because
  - Poorly functioning, small right ventricle
  - Tricuspid regurgitation
  - Variable right ventricular outflow obstruction—abnormal anterior tricuspid valve leaflet. **Therefore, increased right atrial volume shunts blood through foramen ovale or ASD → cyanosis**
- Clinical presentation
  - Severity and presentation depend upon degree of displacement of valve and degree of right ventricular outflow obstruction
    - **May not present until adolescence or adulthood**
    - **If severe in newborn → marked cyanosis, huge heart**
  - **Holosystolic murmur** of tricuspid insufficiency over most of anterior left chest (**most characteristic finding**)
- Diagnosis
  - Chest x-ray—heart size varies from normal to **massive (increased right atrium)**; if severe, **decreased pulmonary blood flow**
  - ECG—tall and broad P waves, right bundle branch block
- Treatment
  - PGE_1
  - Systemic-to-pulmonary shunt
  - Then staged surgery

Note

Patients with Ebstein anomaly may have Wolff-Parkinson-White syndrome (delta wave and short PR interval) and present with episodes of supraventricular tachycardia.

Cyanotic Lesions Associated with Increased Pulmonary Blood Flow

Transposition of the great arteries (TGA)

- Pathophysiology
  - Aorta arises from the right ventricle, and the pulmonary artery from the left ventricle; d = dextroposition of the aorta anterior and the right of the pulmonary artery (normal is posterior and to the right of the pulmonary artery)
  - Series circuit changed to **2 parallel circuits; need foramen ovale and PDA** for some mixture of desaturated and oxygenated blood; better mixing in half of patients with a VSD

Note

Transposition of the Great Arteries

- Most common cyanotic lesion presenting in the immediate newborn period
- More common in infant of diabetic mother

- Clinical presentation
  - **With intact septum (simple TGA)**—as PDA starts to close, severe cyanosis and tachypnea ensue
  - S_2 **usually single and loud;** murmurs absent, or a soft systolic ejection murmur at midleft sternal border
  - If VSD is present, there is a harsh murmur at the lower left sternal border. If large, then holosystolic murmur, significant mixing of blood lessens cyanosis, but presents as heart failure
- Diagnosis
  - Chest x-ray:
    - Mild cardiomegaly, narrow mediastinum, and normal-to-increased pulmonary blood flow
    - **"Egg on a string" appearance**—narrow heart base *plus* absence of main segment of the pulmonary artery
  - ECG—**normal** neonatal right-sided dominance
  - Echocardiogram (gold standard)
- Treatment
  - PGE_1 (keeps PDA patent)
  - Balloon atrial septostomy
  - Arterial switch surgery in first 2 weeks

Truncus Arteriosus

- Pathophysiology
  - **Single arterial trunk arises from the heart and supplies all circulations.**
  - **Truncus overlies a ventral septal defect (always present) and receives blood from both ventricles (total mixing).**
  - Both ventricles are at systemic pressure.
- Clinical presentation
  - With dropping pulmonary vascular resistance in first week of life, **pulmonary blood flow is greatly increased and results in heart failure.**
  - Large volume of pulmonary blood flow with total mixing, **so minimal cyanosis**
  - If uncorrected, **Eisenmenger** physiology
  - **Single truncal valve**, which may be incompetent (high-pitched, early diastolic decrescendo at mid-left sternal border)
  - Initially, **SEM with loud thrill, single S_2, and minimal cyanosis**
  - With decreasing pulmonary vascular resistance (PVR) → **torrential pulmonary blood flow with heart failure;** runoff from truncus to pulmonary circulation → **wide pulse pressure with bounding pulses and hyperdynamic precordium**
  - Apical mid-diastolic rumble (increased flow across mitral valve)
- Diagnosis
  - Chest x-ray—**heart enlargement with increased pulmonary blood flow**
  - ECG—**biventricular hypertrophy**
  - Echocardiogram (gold standard)

Note

Truncus arteriosis is one of the major conotruncal lesions associated with the **CATCH-22** syndrome, i.e., DiGeorge. Also seen are transposition of the great arteries and aortic arch abnormalities.

- Treatment
  - **Treat heart failure**
  - Then surgery in first few weeks of life

MIXED LESIONS

Total Anomalous Pulmonary Venous Return (TAPVR)

- Pathophysiology
  - Complete anomalous drainage of the pulmonary veins into the systemic venous circulation; total mixing of **systemic venous and pulmonary venous blood** within the heart produces cyanosis
  - Right atrial blood → right ventricle and pulmonary artery *or* to left atrium via foramen ovale or ASD
  - **Enlarged right atrium, right ventricle, and pulmonary artery; and small left atrium; and left ventricle normal or small**
- **Clinical manifestations** depend on **presence or absence** of obstruction.
  - **Obstruction (of pulmonary veins, usually infracardiac):**
    - **Severe pulmonary venous congestion and pulmonary hypertension with decreasing cardiac output and shock**
    - Cyanosis and severe tachypnea; may not respond to ventilation and PGE_1 → **need emergent diagnosis and surgery for survival**
    - Heart failure early with mild-to-moderate obstruction and a large left-to-right shunt; pulmonary hypertension and mild cyanosis
  - **No obstruction—total mixing with a large left-to-right shunt; mild cyanosis; less likely to be severely symptomatic early**
- Diagnosis
  - Chest x-ray—large supracardiac shadow with an enlarged cardiac shadow forms a **"snowman" appearance**; pulmonary vascularity is increased
  - ECG—**RVH and tall, spiked P waves (RAE)**
  - Echocardiogram (gold standard)
- Treatment
  - **PGE_1**
  - **Surgical correction**

Note

TAPVR always has an atrial connection.

Hypoplastic Left Heart Syndrome

- Pathophysiology
  - **Atresia of mitral or aortic valves, left ventricle, and ascending aorta (or any combination)**
  - **Right ventricle maintains both pulmonary and systemic circulation.**
  - **Pulmonary venous blood passes through foramen ovale or ASD from left atrium → right atrium and mixes with systemic blood to produce total mixing**
  - Usually, the ventricular septum is intact and all of the right ventricular blood enters the pulmonary artery.

- **Ductus arteriosus supplies the descending aorta, ascending aorta and coronary arteries from retrograde flow.**
- Systemic circulation cannot be maintained, and if there is a **moderate-to-large ASD → pulmonary overcirculation**

- Clinical presentation
  - **Cyanosis may not be evident with ductus open,** but then **gray-blue** skin color (combination of hypoperfusion and cyanosis as ductus closes)
  - **Signs of heart failure, weak or absent pulses, and shock**
  - Enlarged heart with **right parasternal lift;** nondescript systolic murmur
- Diagnosis
  - Chest x-ray—**heart enlargement with increased pulmonary blood flow**
  - ECG—**right ventricular hypertrophy and right arial enlargement with decreased left-sided forces**
  - Echocardiogram (gold standard)
- Treatment
  - **May do nothing** if malformations or genotype not compatible with life
  - The best treatment today is the **three-stage Norwood procedure.** (better results currently than cardiac transplantation)
- Other—many have a significant **abnormality of central nervous system (CNS) and/or kidneys: need careful genetic, neurologic examination and screening tests on any child being considered for surgery**

REGURGITANT LESIONS

Mitral Valve Prolapse

- Abnormal cusps—billowing of one or both leaflets into left atrium toward end of systole (congenital defect)
- Usually not recognizable until adolescence or adulthood; girls > boys
  - May present with chest pain or palpitations
  - Arrhythmias, especially uni- or multifocal premature ventricular contractions
- **Apical late systolic murmur,** preceded by a **click**—in abrupt standing or Valsalva, click may appear earlier in systole and murmur may be more prominent
- Diagnosis
  - ECG—usually normal
  - Chest x-ray—normal
  - Echocardiogram (gold standard)
- No therapy, not progressive; adults (more in men) at risk for cardiovascular complications if have thickened leaflets

Note

Mitral valve prolapse is a common finding in those with Marfan and Ehlers-Danlos syndrome.

OTHER CARDIAC PATHOLOGY

Infective Endocarditis

A 6-year-old boy has had high intermittent fevers for 3 weeks, accompanied by chills. He has a past history of bicuspid aortic valves and recently had dental work.

- Etiology/epidemiology
  - Most are *Streptococcus viridans* (alpha hemolytic) and *Staphylococcus aureus*
  - Organism associations
    - *S. viridans*—after dental procedures
    - Group D streptococci—large bowel or genitourinary manipulation
    - *Pseudomonas aeruginosa* and *Serratia marcescens*—intravenous drug users
    - Fungi—after open heart surgery
    - Coagulase-negative *Staphylococcus*—indwelling intravenous catheters
  - Highest risk with prosthetic valve and uncorrected cyanotic heart lesions
  - Most cases occur after **surgical or dental procedures** (high risk with poor dental hygiene) are performed.
- Clinical presentation
  - **Prolonged intermittent fever, weight loss,** fatigue, myalgia, arthralgia, headache, nausea, vomiting
  - **New or changing heart murmur**
  - Splenomegaly, petechiae, embolic stroke, CNS abscess, CNS hemorrhage, mycotic aneurysm (all more with *Staphylococcus*)
  - Skin findings—rare; late findings (uncommon in treated patients); represent vasculitis from circulating Ag-Ab complexes; if present, are highly suggestive
    - **Osler nodes**—tender, pea-sized, intradermal nodules on pads of fingers and toes
    - **Janeway lesions**—painless, small erythematous or hemorrhagic lesions on palms and soles
    - **Splinter hemorrhage**—linear lesions beneath nail beds
    - **Roth spots**—retinal exudates
- Diagnosis
  - Duke criteria (2 major or 1 major + 3 minor or 5 minor)

Note

Staphylococcal endocarditis is more common in those without underlying heart disease. *Strep viridians* is more common in patients *with* underlying heart disease or after dental procedures.

Table 13-3. Duke Criteria

Major Criteria	Minor Criteria
• **Positive blood culture** (two separate for usual pathogens; at least two for less common) • Evidence on **echocardiogram** (intracardiac or valve lesion, prosthetic regurgitant flow, abscess, partial dehiscence of prosthetic valve, new valvular regurgitant flow)	• Predisposing conditions • Fever • Emboli or vascular signs • Immune complex disease (glomerulo-nephritis, arthritis, positive rheumatoid factor, Osler node, Roth spots [retinal hemorrhages with white centers]) • Single positive blood culture • Echocardiographic signs not meeting criteria

Note

HACEK

- **H**emophilus spp.

- **A**ctinobacillus

- **A**ctinomycetemcomitans

- **C**ardiobacterium hominus

- **E**ikenella corrodens

- **K**ingella kingae

These are slow-growing gram negative organisms that are part of normal flora.

- Complications

  - **Most common—heart failure from aortic or mitral lesions**

  - Others—systemic or pulmonary emboli, myocardial abscess, myocarditis, valve obstruction, heart block, meningitis, osteomyelitis, arthritis, renal abscess, immune complex–mediated glomerulonephritis

- Treatment

  - Organism specific for 4–6 weeks (*S. viridans*, Enterococci, *S. aureus*, MRSA, *S. epidermidis*, HACEK)

  - Heart failure—digitalis, diuretic, salt restriction

  - Surgery—severe aortic or mitral involvement with intractable failure, failure of blood culture to clear, abscess, recurrent emboli, increasing size of vegetations with worsening regurgitation

  - Prophylaxis (AHA, 2007) for:

  - Artifical valves

    ○ Previous history of infective endocarditis

    ○ Unrepaired or incompletely repaired cyanotic disease, including those with palliative shunts and conduits

    ○ A completely repaired defect with prosthetic material or device for first 6 months

    ○ Any residual defect at site of any repair

    ○ Cardiac transplant which develops a problem in a valve

    ○ Given ONLY for dental procedures with manipulation of gingival tissue or peri-apical area or perforation of oral mucosa; incision or biopsy of respiratory tract mucosa and surgery on infected skin or musculoskeletal structures

    ○ Drug of choice is amoxicillin

Acute Rheumatic Fever

A 6-year-old girl complains of severe joint pain in her elbows and wrists. She has had fever for the past 4 days. Past history reveals a sore throat 1 month ago. Physical examination is remarkable for swollen, painful joints and a heart murmur. Laboratory tests show an elevated erythrocyte sedimentation rate and high antistreptolysin (ASO) titers.

- Etiology/epidemiology
  - Related to group A *Streptococcus* infection within several weeks
  - Antibiotics that eliminate *Streptococcus* from pharynx prevent initial episode of acute rheumatic fever
  - Remains **most common form of acquired heart disease worldwide** (but Kawasaki in United States and Japan)
  - Initial attacks and recurrences with peak incidence *Streptococcus* pharyngitis: age 5–15
  - Immune-mediated—antigens shared between certain strep components and mammalian tissues (heart, brain, joint)
- Clinical presentation and diagnosis—Jones criteria. Absolute requirement: evidence of recent *Streptococcus* infection (microbiological or serology); then two major or one major and two minor criteria

Table 13-4. Jones Criteria

Major Criteria	Minor Criteria
Carditis	Fever
Polyarthritis (migratory)	Arthralgia
Erythema marginatum	Elevated acute phase reactants (ESR, CRP)
Chorea	Prolonged PR interval on ECG
Subcutaneous nodules	*Plus* evidence of preceding streptococci infection

Note

If arthritis is present, arthralgia cannot be used as a minor criterion.

The presence of Sydenham's Chorea alone is sufficient for diagnosis.

- Treatment
  - Bed rest and monitor closely
  - **Oral penicillin** or erythromycin (if allergic) for 10 days will eradicate group A strep; then need long-term prophylaxis
  - Anti-inflammatory
    - **Hold if arthritis is only typical manifestation (may interfere with characteristic migratory progression)**
    - Aspirin in patients with arthritis/carditis *without* CHF
    - If carditis with CHF, **prednisone** for 2–3 weeks, then taper; start aspirin for 6 weeks
  - Digoxin, salt restriction, diuretics as needed
  - **If chorea is only isolated finding, do not need aspirin; drug of choice is phenobarbital** (then haloperidol or chlorpromazine)

- Complications
  - Most have no residual heart disease.
  - **Valvular disease most important complication (mitral, aortic, tricuspid)**
- Prevention
  - **Continuous antibiotic prophylaxis**
    - ◦ If carditis—continue into adulthood, perhaps for life; without carditis—lower risk; can discontinue after patient is in their twenties and at least 5 years since last episode
    - ◦ Treatment of choice—**single intramuscular benzathine penicillin G** every 4 weeks
    - ◦ If compliant—penicillin V PO BID or sulfadiazine PO QD; if allergic to both: erythromycin PO BID

Hypertrophic Obstructive Cardiomyopathy (HOCM)

- Pathophysiology
  - **Obstructive left-sided congenital heart disease**
- Decreased compliance, so increased resistance and **decreased left ventricular filling, mitral insufficiency**
- Clinical presentation—weakness, fatigue, dyspnea on exertion, **palpitations, angina, dizziness, syncope; risk of sudden death**
- Cardiovascular examination—**left ventricular lift, no systolic ejection click (differentiates from aortic stenosis),** SEM at left sternal edge and apex (increased after exercise, during Valsalva, and standing)
- Diagnosis
  - ECG—left ventricular hypertrophy ± ST depression and T-wave inversion; may have intracardiac conduction defect
  - Chest x-ray—mild cardiomegaly (prominent LV)
  - Echocardiogram—left ventricular hypertrophy, mostly septal; Doppler—left ventricular outflow gradient usually mid-to-late systole (maximal muscular outflow obstruction)
- Treatment
  - **No competitive sports or strenuous exercise (sudden death)**
  - **Digoxin and aggressive diuresis are contraindicated** (and infusions of other inotropes)
  - **Beta blockers (propranolol) and calcium channel blockers (verapamil)**

Note

Suspect hypertrophic cardiopathy in an athlete with sudden death.

HYPERTENSION

A 5-year-old girl is noted to have blood pressure above the 95th percentile on routine physical examination. The rest of the examination is unremarkable. Her blood pressure remains elevated on repeat measurement over the next few weeks. Past history is remarkable for a treated urinary tract infection 1 year ago. Complete blood cell count is normal; urinalysis is normal. Blood urea nitrogen is 24 mg/dL and creatinine is 1.8 mg/dL.

Note

When a child presents with hypertension, think of renal causes.

- Routine blood pressure check beginning at 3 years of age
  - If increased blood pressure, check all 4 extremities (coarctation)
  - Normal—blood pressure in legs should be 10–20 mm Hg higher than in arms
- Blood pressure increases with age—need standard nomograms
  - If mild hypertension, repeat twice over next 6 weeks
  - If consistently >95% for age, need further evaluation
- Etiology—essential (primary) or secondary
  - Secondary—**most common in infants and younger children**
    - Newborn—umbilical artery catheters → renal artery thrombosis
    - Early childhood—renal disease, coarctation, endocrine, medications
    - Adolescent—essential hypertension
  - **Renal and renovascular hypertension—majority of causes may be due to urinary tract infection** (secondary to an obstructive lesion), acute glomerulonephritis, Henoch-Schönlein purpura with nephritis, hemolytic uremic syndrome, acute tubular necrosis, renal trauma, leukemic infiltrates, mass lesions, renal artery stenosis
  - Essential hypertension—more common in adults and adolescents
    - Positive family history
    - Multifactorial—obesity, genetic, and physiologic changes
- Diagnosis
  - CBC, blood chemistries, UA, ECG, echo, renal ultrasound, angiogram (less common)
- Treatment
  - If obese—weight control, aerobic exercise, no-added-salt diet, monitor blood pressure
  - Pharmacologic treatment (secondary hypertension and selective primary)—similar use of drugs as in adults

Gastrointestinal Disease 14

Learning Objectives

❏ Demonstrate understanding of disorders of the oral cavity

❏ Diagnose and describe treatments for children who present with gastroenteritis, vomiting, hematochezia, or constipation

ORAL CAVITY

Cleft Lip and Palate

- Most are **multifactorial** inheritance; also **autosomal dominant in families (most with isolated cleft palate)**
- Clefts are highest among Asians, lowest among African descent
- **Increase in other malformations with isolated cleft palate**
- **Most important early issue is feeding (special nipple needed)**
- Complications—increased risk of otitis media, hearing loss, speech problems
- Treatment—surgical correction
  - Lip at 3 months of age
  - Palate at <1 year

GASTROENTERITIS

Acute Diarrhea

A 13-month-old child has had a 3-day history of green watery stools. She has also been vomiting for 1 day. Physical examination reveals a febrile, irritable baby with dry mucous membranes and sunken eyes.

- Etiology (*see* Table 14-1)

Table 14-1. Causes of Diarrhea (Acute and Chronic)

	Infant	Child	Adolescent
Acute	• Gastroenteritis • Systemic infection • Antibiotic	• Gastroenteritis/Food poisoning • Systemic infection	• Gastroenteritis/food poisoning • Systemic infection
Chronic	• Postinfectious lactase deficiency • Milk/soy intolerance • Chronic diarrhea of infancy • Celiac disease • Cystic fibrosis	• Postinfectious lactase deficiency • Irritable bowel syndrome • Celiac disease • Lactose intolerance • *Giardiasis* • Inflammatory bowel disease	• Irritable bowel syndrome • Inflammatory bowel disease • Lactose intolerance • *Giardiasis* • Laxative abuse

- Common organisms (*see* Table 14-2)

Table 14-2. Common Causes of Acute Diarrhea

Bacterial (Inflammatory)	Viral	Parasitic
Campylobacter	**Norovirus**	*Giardia lamblia* (most common)
Enteroinvasive *E. coli*	Rotavirus	*E. histolytica*
Salmonella	Enteric adenovirus	*Strongyloides*
Shigella	Astrovirus	*Balantidium coli*
Yersinia	Calicivirus	*Cryptosporidium parvum*
Clostridium difficile		*Trichuris trichiura*
E. coli 0157:H7		

- Major transmission is **fecal/oral** or by **ingestion of contaminated food or water**
- Clinical presentation
  - Diarrhea, vomiting, abdominal cramps, nausea, fever (suggests inflammation and dehydration)
  - Can present from an **extraintestinal infection**, e.g., urinary tract infection, pneumonia, hepatitis
- Management
  - **Assess hydration and provide fluid and electrolyte replacement**
  - Prevent spread
  - In some cases, determine etiology and provide specific therapy (some are not treated)
  - Think about **daycare** attendance, recent **travel,** use of **antibiotics,** exposures, intake of **seafood, unwashed vegetables, unpasteurized milk, contaminated water, uncooked meats to isolate differential diagnosis of organisms**
- Labs
  - Most cost-effective, noninvasive testing is **stool examination**

- Mucus, blood, leukocytes → colitis (invasive or cytotoxic organism)
- Stool cultures—with blood, leukocytes, suspected hemolytic uremic syndrome, immunosuppressed, in outbreaks
- *Clostridium difficile* toxin—if recent history of antibiotics
- Ova and parasites
- Enzyme immunoassays for viruses or PCR (rarely need to be diagnosed)

Chronic Diarrhea

Table 14-3. Organism-Specific Associations and Therapy

Organism	Association	Therapy
Rotavirus	Watery diarrhea, vomiting, ± fever	Supportive
Enteropathogenic *E. coli*	Nurseries, daycare	Supportive care in severe cases, neomycin or colistin
Enterotoxigenic *E. coli*	Traveler's diarrhea	Supportive care trimetho prim-sulfamethoxazole in severe cases
Enterhemorrhagic *E. coli*	Hemorrhagic colitis, HUS	**No antimicrobial therapy** in suspected cases due to ↑ risk of HUS; supportive care only
Salmonella	Infected animals and contaminated eggs, milk, poultry	Treatment indicated *only* for patients who are ≤3 months of age, toxic, has disseminated disease, or *S. typhi*
Shigella	Person-to-person spread, contaminated food	Trimethoprim/sulfamethoxazole
Campylobacter	Person-to-person spread, contaminated food	Self-limiting; erythromycin speeds recovery and reduces carrier state; recommended for severe disease
Yersinia enterocolitica	Pets, contaminated food, arthritis, rash	No antibiotic therapy; aminoglycosides plus a third-generation cephalosporin for infants ≤3 months of age or with culture-proven septicemia
Clostridium difficile	History of antibiotic use	Metronidazole or vancomycin and discontinuation of other antibiotics
Staphylococcus aureus	Food poisoning (onset within 12 h of ingestion)	Supportive care, antibiotics rarely indicated
Entamoeba histolytica	Acute blood diarrhea	Metronidazole
Giardia	Anorexia, nausea, abdominal distension, watery diarrhea, weight loss Cysts ingested from infected individual or from contaminated food or water	Metronidazole, furazolidone
Cryptosporidium	Mild diarrhea in immuno-compromised infants; severe diarrhea in AIDS patients	Raising CD4 count to normal is best treatment. No proven therapy (antimicrobial); strong supportive care; may try rifabutin

Definition of abbreviations: HUS, hemolytic uremia syndrome

Chronic Diarrhea and Malabsorption

- Patterns
  - From birth
  - After introduction of a new food
- Clinical presentation
  - Chronic nonspecific diarrhea of infancy:
    - **Weight, height, and nutritional status is normal, and no fat in stool**
    - Excessive intake of fruit juice, carbonated fluids, low fat intake usually present in history
  - Diarrhea with carbohydrates—CHO malabsorption
  - Weight loss and stool with high fat—think malabsorption
- Workup of chronic diarrhea (simple, noninvasive testing to be done first)
  - History and physical, nutritional assessment; **stool** for pH, reducing substances, fat, blood, leukocytes, culture, *C. difficile* toxin, ova, and parasites
  - Blood studies—complete blood count and differential, ESR, electrolytes, glucose, BUN, and creatinine
  - **Sweat test, 72-hour fecal fat,** breath hydrogen tests
- Initial evaluation
  - Fat:
    - **Most useful screening test is stool for fat (Sudan red stain)**
    - **Confirm with 72-hour stool for fecal fat (gold standard for steatorrhea)**
    - **Steatorrhea is most prominent with pancreatic insufficiency; all require a sweat chloride**
    - Serum trypsinogen is also a good screen (reflects residual pancreatic function)
  - CHO malabsorption—screen with **reducing substances in stool (Clinitest)**
    - **Breath hydrogen test**—after a known CHO load, the collected breath hydrogen is analyzed and malabsorption of the specific CHO is identified
  - Protein loss—cannot be evaluated directly (large proportion of bacterial protein and dietary protein almost completely absorbed before terminal ileum; amino acids and peptides are reabsorbed)
    - Screen—**spot stool α_1-antitrypsin level**
- More common differential diagnosis of malabsorption
  - **Giardiasis—only common primary infection causing chronic malabsorption; duodenal aspirate/biopsy/immunoassay (Giardia)**
  - HIV or congenital T- or B-cell defects
  - Small-bowel disease—**gluten enteropathy**, abetalipoproteinemia, lymphangiectasia
  - Pancreatic insufficiency—fat malabsorption (**cystic fibrosis is most common congenital disorder associated with malabsorption)**
  - Most common anomaly causing incomplete bowel obstruction with malabsorption is **malrotation**
  - **Short bowel**—congenital or postnatal loss of >50% of small bowel with or without a portion of the large intestine (presence of ileocecal valve is better)
  - **Celiac disease**—associated with exposure to **gluten** (rye, wheat, barley, derivatives)

- Patients mostly age 6 months to 2 years
- **Permanent intolerance**
- Genetic predisposition (HLA DQ2)
- Clinical presentation
- Diarrhea
- Failure to thrive
- Growth retardation
- Vomiting
- Anorexia, not interested in feeding
- Ataxia
- Evaluation
  - Blood for anti-tissue transglutaminase (IgA) and serum IgA (false if IgA deficiency) (best initial test)
  - Definitive test—small intestine biopsy
- Treatment—**lifelong, strict gluten-free diet**

VOMITING

Esophageal Atresia (EA) and Tracheoesophageal Fistula (TEF)

- Three basic types:
  - Isolated EA
  - Isolated (H-type) TEF
  - EA and distal TEF
- Most common anatomy is **upper esophagus ends in blind pouch and TEF connected to distal esophagus**
- **H-type—presents chronically** and diagnosed later in life with chronic respiratory problems
- Half with associated anomalies—**VACTERL** association
- Clinical presentation in neonate (EA or EA + TEF)
  - **Frothing, bubbling, cough, cyanosis, and respiratory distress**
  - **With feedings → immediate regurgitation and aspiration**
- Clinical presentation with just TEF—feeding problems and recurrent aspiration
- Diagnosis
  - **Inability to pass nasogastric/orogastric tube**
  - Esophageal atresia: x-ray shows coiled nasogastric tube in blind pouch with no distal gas (gasless abdomen)
  - **Isolated** TEF: **esophagram with contrast media** (or bronchoscopy or endoscopy with methylene blue)
  - Esophageal atresia and distal fistula: coiled nasogastric tube in blind pouch the large amount of air in stomach and intestines
- Treatment—surgical ligation of TEF and resection with end-to-end anastomosis of esophageal atresia

Note

VACTERL Association

Nonrandom association of birth defects:

Vertebral anomalies

Anal atresia

Cardiac defect

Tracheo**E**sophageal fistula

Renal anamolies

Limb abnormalities

Gastroesophageal Reflux Disease (GERD)

A 4-month-old is admitted with episodes of apnea occurring 20–30 min after feeds. The mother states the baby has been spitting up since birth. She is at the fifth percentile for weight.

- Etiology—insufficient lower esophageal sphincter tone early in life
- Symptoms during first few months of life; **resolves by 12–24 months of age;** in older children—chronic (more like adults); only half resolve completely
- Clinical presentation
  - **Postprandial regurgitation**
  - Signs of **esophagitis**—arching, **irritability,** feeding aversion, failure to thrive
  - **Obstructive apnea,** stridor, **lower airway disease (cough, wheezing)**
- Diagnosis
  - Most by history and physical
  - **Barium esophagram and upper gastrointestinal studies**
  - **Esophageal pH monitoring (best test)**—quantitative and sensitive documentation of acid reflux (normal pH in lower esophagus is <4 only 5–8% of time)
  - **Endoscopy**—**erosive esophagitis** and complications
  - Radionucleotide scintigraphy (Tc)—to document aspiration
  - Laryngotracheobronchoscopy—for extraesophageal GERD
- Management
  - **Conservative** with lifestyle management: normalize **feeding technique, appropriate volume, thicken feeds, positioning**
  - Pharmacologic:
    - **H₂-receptor antagonist** (ranitidine, cimetidine, famotidine)—**first-line** with overall best safety profile
    - **Proton pump inhibitor** (omeprazole, lansoprazole, pantoprazole)—most potent for severe reflux and esophagitis
  - Surgery—**fundoplication** for refractory esophagitis, strictures, chronic pulmonary disease, continued obstructive apnea

Pyloric Stenosis

A 4-week-old boy has nonbilious projectile vomiting. Physical examination is remarkable for a small mass palpated in the abdomen.

- Epidemiology—more common in whites of Northern European ancestry, **firstborn males**
- Clinical presentation
  - **Nonbilious, projectile vomiting**
  - **Still hungry and desire to feed more**
  - Usually age ≥3 weeks (1 week to 5 months)

Note

Prokinetic agents (metaclopramide, bethanechol or erythromycin) have no efficacy in the treatment of GERD in children.

Note

Pyloric stenosis is high yield for the exam.

- – Mild-to-moderate dehydration, **hypochloremic, hypokalemic metabolic alkalosis**
- – Palpation of a firm, movable, 2-cm, **olive-shaped,** hard mass in midepigastrium; left to right peristaltic wave
- Diagnosis—best test is **ultrasound** (a target-like appearance in cross-section)
- Treatment
  - – Rehydrate, correct electrolytes (NaCl, KCl)
  - – **Pyloromyotomy**

Duodenal Atresia

A newborn presents with bilious vomiting with every feed. Abdominal film reveals a double bubble.

- Epidemiology
  - – Half are born premature
  - – **Down syndrome**
  - – With other anomalies—malrotation, esophageal atresia, congenital heart defects, anorectal malformation, renal anomalies
- Clinical presentation
  - – **Bilious vomiting *without* abdominal distention on first day of life** (obstruction just distal to ampulla)
  - – **Polyhydramnios** prenatally
  - – Many with **jaundice** (increased enterohepatic circulation)
- Diagnosis
  - – X-ray shows classic **double bubble with *no* distal bowel gas.**
  - – X-ray spine for anomalies; ultrasound for other anomalies
- Treatment
  - – **Nasogastric decompression**
  - – Intravenous fluids
  - – **Surgery**—duodenoduodenostomy

Note

Jejunal or Ileal Atresia

Most present on the first day of life.

There is bile-stained emesis with abdominal distention. (With duodenal atresia, there is no abdominal distention.)

Plain films show air-fluid levels.

Contrast studies of the upper and lower intestine can delineate level of obstruction.

Ultrasound may also differentiate intestinal atresia from meconium ileus from malrotation.

Table 14-4. Congenital Bowel Obstruction

Lesion	Etiology	DDX	Clinical Background/ Presentation	Diagnosis	Management Algorithm/ Definitive Treatment
Duodenal Atresia	Failed recanalization of bowel lumen 4th–7th week gestation	• Duodenal stenosis • Annular pancreas • Duplication cysts • Ladd bands from malrotation	• Polyhydramnios • 50% premature • Other organ system anomalies • Half with chromosomal anomalies, especially trisomy 21 **Presentation** • First day • Bilious vomiting w/o abdominal distention • Jaundice	• **Prenatal sonogram** • **Postnatal plain X-ray:** double-bubble with NO distal bowel gas • **CXR, spine films** • **Echocardiogram** • **Renal ultrasound** for other most common anomalies	• NG/OG decompression • NPO + IV fluids + electrolyte balance • Broad-spectrum antibiotics **Definitive Treatment:** **Surgery when stable—**duodenoduodenostomy
Jejunal and Ileal Atresias	Intrauterine vascular accident → segmental infarction and resorption of fetal intestine	• Meconium ileus/ plug • Malrotation ± volvulus • Hirschprung disease	• Possible role with antenatal cigarette and/or cocaine use • Very little familial inheritance (aut. rec.) • Little extraintestinal anomalies **Presentation** • Polyhydramnios • Abdominal distention at birth or with first feeds + vomiting, may be bilious • Few with delayed or no passage of meconium • Jaundice	• Less likely to be detected in utero • **Plain X-ray:** multiple air-fluid levels proximal to obstruction in upright or lateral decubitus • **Ultrasound:** differentiate with meconium ileus and identify malrotation • **Contrast studies** to localize	• NG/OG • IV fluid and electrolyte balance prior to surgery • Antibiotics **Definitive Treatment:** **Surgery—**resect dilated proximal bowel then end-to-end anastamosis

(Continued)

Table 14-4. Congenital Bowel Obstruction (*Continued*)

Lesion	Etiology	DDX	Clinical Background/ Presentation	Diagnosis	Management Algorithm/ Definitive Treatment
Meconium Ileus	Abnormal viscous secretions → distal 20-30 cm of ileum collapsed and proximal bowel dilated and filled with thick meconium impacted in ileum	• Meconium plug • Atresias • Hirschprung disease • Malrotation ± volvulus	• 80-90% will be diagnosed with CF • May perforate in utero → meconium peritonitis (calcifications) **Presentation:** • Vomiting becomes persistent with prominent abdominal distention • No passage of meconium • May present as bowel perforation and peritonitis • Palpation of "doughy" or cordlike masses	• **Plain films:** dilated loops of bowel proximal to obstruction that vary with width and not evenly filled with gas • Presence of bubbly or granular appearance in RLQ (meconium with gas bubbles) • No air-fluid levels as secretions are too viscid to layer • **Ultrasound** to verify if questionable • **Water-soluble enema** (Gastrografin or Hypaque) will localize • **Test for CF**	• NPO • NG/OG decompression • IV fluid and electrolyte balance • Antibiotics **Definitive Treatment:** **First:** hypertonic water-soluble contrast enema to attempt wash-out **If fails**—laparotomy
Meconium Plugs	Decreased water content for many possible reasons leads to lower colonic or anorectal meconium plug	• Meconium ileus • Hirschprung disease	• Majority not associated with CF, unless in small bowel • Infants with polycythemia, dehydration and small left colon as may be seen with IODM • Maternal opiate use or treatment with MgSO4 **Presentation:** Failure of meconium passage and abdominal distention	• **Plain films:** low obstruction with proximal bowel dilatation and multiple air-fluid levels	• NG/OG + NPO • IV fluid and electrolyte balance • Antibiotics **Definitive Treatment:** • Evacuation with glycerin suppository if very low or saline enema or hypertonic water-soluble contrast if higher • Observe for possible Hirschprung disease • Consider sweat test if contrast shows small bowel plug.

(*Continued*)

Table 14-4. Congenital Bowel Obstruction (*Continued*)

Lesion	Etiology	DDX	Clinical Background/ Presentation	Diagnosis	Management Algorithm/ Definitive Treatment

Malrotation	• As developing bowel rotates in and out of abdominal cavity (weeks 5-12), superior mesenteric artery acts as the axis
	
	• With nonrotation, 1st and 2nd part of duodenum are in normal position, but because of inadequate mesenteric attachment to posterior wall, rest of small bowel occupies RLQ and colon the left
	
	• Failure of cecum to move to the RLQ → failure to form broad-based adhesions to posterior wall → superior mesenteric artery is tethered by a narrow stalk (causes volvulus) and Ladd bands can extend from cecum to RUQ and obstruct at duodenum.
		• Intestinal atresias
		• Meconium ileus
		• Hirschprung disease
			• Other anomalies of abdominal wall
			  – Diaphragmatic hernia
			  – Gastroschisis
			  – Omphalocele
			  – Heterotaxy syndrome (CHD, malrotation, asplenia/ polysplenia)
			
			Presentation:
			• 1st year of life with > 50% in first month with symptoms due to intermittent volvulus and/ or Ladd band obstruction -acute and chronic obstruction (recurrent pain and vomiting)
			• Can present in first week with bilious emesis and acute obstruction
			• May have, malabsorption due to bacterial overgrowth
			• Any age with acute obstruction due to volvulus
				• **Plain film:** may show double-bubble with evidence of small amount of distal gas (prior to the volvulus) or a gasless abdomen
				• **Ultrasound:** inversion of superior mesenteric artery and vein
				• **Upper GI:** malposition of ligament of Treitz and small bowel obstruction with corkscrew appearance or duodenal obstruction with "bird's beak" appearance
					• **If volvulus:** emergency surgery after IV and fluids
					• Otherwise NPO, NG/ OG
					• Correct fluid and electrolyte imbalance.
					
					Definitive Treatment:
					• **Surgery:** any patient of any age with any significant rotational abnormality
					• **Volvulus:** acute surgical emergency

(*Continued*)

Table 14-4. Congenital Bowel Obstruction (*Continued*)

Lesion	Etiology	DDX	Clinical Background/ Presentation	Diagnosis	Management Algorithm/ Definitive Treatment
Hirschprung Disease	• Developmental disorder of the enteric nervous system such that there are absence of ganglion cells in the submucosal and myenteric plexus • Arrest of neuroblast migration from proximal to distal bowel → inadequate relaxation and hypertonicity	• Long segment disease vs., intestinal atresia • Meconium plug • Meconium ileus	• Most common cause of intestinal obstruction in neonate • Usual short segment is male preponderance but equalizes with long segment disease • Increased familial incidence with long segment but must (short segment) are sporadic • May be associated with cardiovascular and urological defects and with Down syndrome • 80% are short (rectosigmoid) • 10-15% long (more than that) • 5% total bowel aganglionosis **Presentation:** • Most diagnosed in neonates • Suspect with any delayed meconium passage in full term infant (99% within first 48 hours) or no passage with progressive abdominal distension and vomiting • Later with chronic constipation and empty rectum on digital exam with subsequent explosive release of small stool and gas • Main concern is meconium enterocolitis	• **Plain film:** distended loops of bowel • **Contrast enema** may not show classic line of demarcation form small aganglionic bowel to proximal dilatation (better >1 month of age) but 24 hr films usually show retained contrast and suggests the diagnosis • **Barium enema** also useful prior to surgery to define extent of aganglionic segment • **Gold standard confirmation is the suction rectal biopsy**	• NG/OG • NPO • Fluid and electrolyte management • Evaluate for other defects **Definitive Treatment:** Laparoscopic single-stage endorectal pull-through is procedure of choice.

Note

A delay in treating volvulus can result in short bowel syndrome.

Malrotation and Volvulus

- Etiology
  - **Incomplete rotation of intestine during fetal development**
  - Superior mesenteric artery acts as axis for rotation
  - **Ladd bands may extend from cecum to right upper quadrant (RUQ) to produce duodenal obstruction**
- Clinical presentation
  - Most present in first year of life with acute or chronic incomplete obstruction
  - **Bilious emesis, recurrent abdominal pain with vomiting**
  - **An acute small-bowel obstruction in a patient without previous bowel surgery is suspicious for volvulus (acute surgical abdomen)**
- Diagnosis
  - Plain film is nonspecific—may show double bubble if there is duodenal obstruction
  - Barium enema shows malposition of cecum (mobile cecum is not situated in the right lower quadrant); upper gastrointestinal will show malposition of ligament of Treitz
  - **Ultrasound will show inversion of superior mesenteric artery and vein (superior mesenteric vein to the left of the artery is suggestive) and duodenal obstruction with thickened bowel loops to the right of the spine; advantage is no need for contrast; start with this study**
- Treatment—surgery

HEMATOCHEZIA

Meckel Diverticulum

Note

Meckel diverticulum: "Disease of 2s"

- 2 years of age
- 2% of population
- 2 types of tissue
- 2 inches in size
- 2 ft from ileocecal valve

A 2-year-old boy presents with a 1-week history of painless rectal bleeding. Physical examination is unremarkable. The abdomen is soft and nontender. Rectal examination is unremarkable.

- Etiology
  - Remnant of embryonic yolk sac (omphalomesenteric or vitelline duct), **lining similar to stomach**
  - **Most frequent congenital gastrointestinal anomaly**
- Clinical presentation
  - Acid-secreting mucosa causes **intermittent painless rectal bleeding**
  - May get anemia, but blood loss is self-limited
  - May have partial or complete bowel obstruction (lead point for an intussusception) or develop diverticulitis and look like acute appendicitis (much less common presentation)
- Diagnosis—**Meckel radionuclide scan** (Tc-99m pertechnetate)
- Treatment—**surgical excision**

Intussusception

A 15-month-old child is seen for cramping, colicky abdominal pain of 12 h duration. He has had two episodes of vomiting and a fever. Physical examination is remarkable for a lethargic child; abdomen is tender to palpation. Leukocytosis is present. During examination, the patient passes a bloody stool with mucus.

- Etiology
  - **Telescoping** of bowel; most **ileal-colic**
  - Most present at age 3 months to 6 years (80% <2 years)
  - Commonly **following adenovirus or rotavirus** infection, upper respiratory infection, otitis media
  - Associated with HSP (Henoch-Schönlein purpura)
  - Can also occur with a **leading point**—Meckel diverticulum, polyp, neurofibroma, hemangioma, malignancy
- Pathophysiology—bowel drags mesentery with it and produces arterial and venous obstruction and mucosal necrosis → classic **"black currant jelly" stool**
- Clinical presentation
  - **Sudden onset of severe paroxysmal colicky abdominal pain; straining, legs flexed**
  - **Progressive weakness**
  - **Lethargy, shock with fever**
  - Vomiting in most (early on, it is bile-stained)
  - Decreased stooling
  - Blood in most patients in first 12 hours, but may be delayed or not at all
- Physical examination—slightly tender, **sausage-shaped mass on right in cephalocaudal axis**
- Diagnosis
  - Ultrasound to first screen for the diagnosis (non-invasive and cost-effective; "doughnut appearance") and look for free-air (if intussusception has caused perforation)
  - Air enema is the next study of choice as it is far safer than the previously-used barium enema (0.1 vs. 2.5% risk of perforation); air enema may be therapeutic and prevent the need for immediate surgery
- Treatment
  - If prolonged, shock, peritoneal irritation, or perforation → surgery
  - **Radiographic reduction under fluoroscopy**—most will reduce if done within 48 hours of presentation (goes down to half after that time)
  - If surgical—**if manual operative reduction is not possible or bowel is not viable, then resection and end-to-end anastomosis**

Note

Other causes of GI bleed

- Anal fissure (most common cause of lower GI bleed in infancy)

- Accidental swallowing of maternal blood (do Apt test)

- Peptic ulcer disease

CONSTIPATION

Functional Constipation

A 6-year-old boy complains of hard bowel movements every fifth day. Physical examination reveals normal weight and height. Abdomen is soft, and hard stool is palpable on rectal examination.

- Delay or difficulty in stooling for at least 2 weeks; typically after age 2 years
- Passage of painful bowel movements with **voluntary withholding** to avoid pain
- May have blood in stool
- Physical examination—**large volume of stool palpated in suprapubic area; rectal exam shows vault filled with stool**
- Treatment
  - Patient education (**bowel training program**)
  - **Relief of impaction**—enema, then stool softeners (mineral oil, lactulose, polyethylene glycol; no prolonged use of stimulants)
  - Behavioral modification
  - Deal with any psychosocial issues

Hirschsprung Disease

- Etiology—absence of a ganglion cells in bowel wall beginning at internal anal sphincter and extending variably proximally
- **Most common reason for bowel obstruction in neonates**
- Clinical presentation
  - Symptoms usually present at birth
  - **Suspect in any full-term infant with a delay in passage of meconium (>24 hours)**
  - May have subsequent history of chronic constipation (if short aganglionic segment)
- Diagnosis
  - Rectal manometry
  - Rectal suction biopsy is definitive
  - Presence of **transition zone** on barium enema (not necessary to perform)
- Treatment—**surgery** (most with temporary colostomy) and wait 6–12 months for definitive correction (most achieve continence)
- Complications—enterocolitis

Table 14-5. Functional Constipation Versus Hirschsprung Disease

	Functional Constipation	**Hirschsprung Disease**
Onset constipation	After 2 years of age	At birth
Failure to thrive	Uncommon	Possible
Enterocolitis	No	Possible
Abdominal distention	Usually not	Yes
Poor weight gain	Usually not	Common
Anal tone	Normal	Normal
Rectal	Stool in ampulla	No stool
Anorectal manometry	Distention of rectum → relaxation of internal sphincter	No sphincter relaxation
Barium enema	Large amount of stool; no transition zone	Transition zone with delayed evacuation

Renal and Urologic Disorders 15

Learning Objectives

❏ Recognize and describe treatment for urinary tract infection, vesicoureteral reflux, obstructive uropathy, and polycystic kidney disease

❏ Diagnose and describe treatments for disorders presenting with hematuria or proteinuria

URINARY TRACT INFECTION (UTI)

A 12-day-old infant presents with fever of 39°C (102°F), vomiting, and diarrhea. On physical examination, the infant appears to be ill and mildly dehydrated.

- Epidemiology—UTI more common in boys than in girls until after second year
- Etiology—colonic bacteria (mostly *E. coli*, then *Klebsiella* and *Proteus*; some *S. saprophyticus*)
- Types
  - *Cystitis*—dysuria, urgency, frequency, suprapubic pain, incontinence, **no fever** (unless very young)
  - *Pyelonephritis*—**abdominal or flank pain, fever, malaise, nausea, vomiting, diarrhea; nonspecific in newborns and infants**
  - *Asymptomatic bacteriuria*—positive urine culture without signs or symptoms; can become symptomatic if untreated; almost exclusive to girls
- Risk factors
  - Females:
    - ◦ Wiping
    - ◦ Sexual activity
    - ◦ Pregnancy
  - Males—uncircumcised
  - Both:
    - ◦ **Vesicoureteral reflux**
    - ◦ Toilet-training
    - ◦ Constipation
    - ◦ **Anatomic abnormalities**

- Diagnosis—**urine culture (gold standard)**—and UA findings
  - Need a proper sample—**if toilet-trained, midstream collection; otherwise, supra-pubic tap or catheterization**
  - Positive if >50,000 colonies/mL (single pathogen) plus pyuria
- Treatment
  - Lower-urinary tract infection (cystitis) with amoxicillin, **trimethoprim-sulfa-methoxazole, or nitrofurantoin** (if no fever)
  - **Pyelonephritis** start with oral antibiotics, unless patient requires hospitalization and IV fluids
- Follow up
  - **Do urine culture** 1 week after stopping antibiotics to confirm sterility; periodic reassessment for next 1–2 years
  - **Obtain ultrasound** for anatomy, suspected abscess, hydronephrosis, recurrent UTI
  - **Obtain voiding cystourethrogram** (VCUG) in recurrent UTIs or UTIs with complications or abnormal ultrasound findings

VESICOURETERAL REFLUX (VUR)

A 2-year-old girl presents with urinary tract infection. She has had multiple urinary tract infections since birth but has never had any follow-up studies to evaluate these infections. Physical examination is remarkable for an ill-appearing child who has a temperature of 40°C (104°F) and is vomiting.

- Definition—abnormal backflow of urine from bladder to kidney
- Etiology
  - Occurs when the submucosal tunnel between the mucosa and detrusor muscle is short or absent.
  - **Predisposition to pyelonephritis → scarring → reflux nephropathy (hypertension, proteinuria, renal insufficiency to end-stage renal disease [ESRD], impaired kidney growth)**
- Grading
  - *Grade I:* into nondilated ureter (common for anyone)
  - *Grade II:* upper collecting system without dilatation
  - *Grade III:* into dilated collecting system with calyceal blunting
  - *Grade IV:* grossly dilated ureter and ballooning of calyces
  - *Grade V:* massive; significant dilatation and tortuosity of ureter; intrarenal reflux with blunting of renal pedicles
- Diagnosis
  - **VCUG for diagnosis and grading**
  - **Renal scan for renal size, scarring and function; if scarring, follow creatinine**
- Natural history
  - Increased scarring with grade 5 (less so with bilateral 4)
  - Majority < grade 5 resolve regardless of age at diagnosis or whether it is unilateral or bilateral
  - With growth, tendency to resolve (lower > higher grades); resolve by age 6–7 years

- Treatment
  - Medical—based on reflux resolving over time; most problems can be taken care of **nonsurgically**
  - Careful ongoing monitoring for and aggressive treatment of all UTIs
  - Surgery if medical therapy fails, if grade 5 reflux, or if any worsening on VCUG or renal scan

OBSTRUCTIVE UROPATHY

- Definition—obstruction of urinary outflow tract
- Clinical presentation
  - **Hydronephrosis**
  - Upper abdominal or flank pain
  - Pyelonephritis, UTI (recurrent)
  - Weak, decreased urinary stream
  - Failure to thrive, diarrhea (or other nonspecific symptoms)
- Diagnosis
  - **Palpable abdominal mass in newborn; most common cause is hydronephrosis,,** due to ureteropelvic junction obstruction or **multicystic kidney disease** (less so–infantile polycystic disease)
  - **Most can be diagnosed prenatally with ultrasound.**
  - **Obtain VCUG in all cases of congenital hydronephrosis and in any with ureteral dilatation to rule out posterior urethral valves**
- Common etiologies
  - **Ureteropelvic junction obstruction—most common** (unilateral or bilateral hydronephrosis)
  - Ectopic ureter—drains outside bladder; causes continual incontinence and UTIs
  - Ureterocele—cystic dilatation with obstruction from a pinpoint ureteral orifice; mostly in girls
  - **Posterior urethral valves:**
    - **Most common cause of severe obstructive uropathy; mostly in boys**
    - **Can lead to end-stage renal disease**
    - **Present with mild hydronephrosis to severe renal dysplasia; suspect in a male with a palpable, distended bladder and weak urinary stream**
- Diagnosis—voiding cystourethrogram (VCUG)
- Treatment
  - Decompress bladder with catheter
  - Antibiotics (intravenously)
  - Transurethral ablation or vesicostomy
- Complications
  - If lesion is severe, may present with pulmonary hypoplasia (Potter sequence)
  - Prognosis dependent on lesion severity and recovery of renal function

DISEASES PRESENTING PRIMARILY WITH HEMATURIA

Acute Poststreptococcal Glomerulonephritis

A 10-year-old boy presents with Coca-Cola–colored urine and edema of his lower extremities. On physical examination, the patient has a blood pressure of 185/100 mm Hg. He does not appear to be in any distress. His lungs are clear to auscultation, and his heart has a regular rate and rhythm without any murmurs, gallops, or rubs. His past medical history is remarkable for a sore throat that was presumed viral by his physician 2 weeks before.

- Etiology
  - **Follows infection with nephrogenic strains of group A beta-hemolytic streptococci of the throat (mostly in cold weather) or skin (in warm weather)**
  - Diffuse mesangial cell proliferation with an increase in mesangial matrix; **lumpy-bumpy deposits of immunoglobulin (Ig) and complement** on glomerular basement membrane and in mesangium
  - Mediated by immune mechanisms but complement activation is mostly through the alternate pathway
- Clinical presentation
  - Most 5–12 years old (corresponds with typical age for strep throat)
  - **1–2 weeks after strep pharyngitis or 3–6 weeks after skin infection (impetigo)**
  - Ranges from asymptomatic microscopic hematuria to acute renal failure
  - **Edema, hypertension, hematuria (classic triad)**
  - Constitutional symptoms—malaise, lethargy, fever, abdominal or flank pain
- Diagnosis
  - Urinalysis—RBCs, **RBC casts**, protein 1–2 +, polymorphonuclear cells
  - Mild normochromic anemia (hemodilution and low-grade hemolysis)
  - **Low C3** (returns to normal in 6–8 weeks)
  - **Need positive throat culture or increasing antibody titer to streptococcal antigens; best single test is the anti-DNase antigen**
  - Consider biopsy only in presence of acute renal failure, nephrotic syndrome, absence of streptococcal or normal complement; or if present >2 months after onset
- Complications
  - Hypertension
  - Acute renal failure
  - Congestive heart failure
  - Electrolyte abnormalities
  - Acidosis
  - Seizures
  - Uremia
- Treatment (in-patient, if severe)
  - Antibiotics for 10 days (penicillin)
  - Sodium restriction, diuresis

Note

For diagnosis of prior Strep infection, use streptozyme (slide agglutination), which detects antibodies to streptolysin O, DNase B, hyaluronidase, streptokinase, and nicotinamide-adenine dinucleotidase.

- Fluid and electrolyte management
- Control hypertension (calcium channel blocker, vasodilator, or angiotensin-converting enzyme inhibitor)
- Complete recovery in >95%

Other Glomerulonephritides

IgA Nephropathy (Berger disease)

- **Most common chronic glomerular disease worldwide**
- Clinical presentation
  - Most commonly presents with gross hematuria **in association with upper respiratory infection** or gastrointestinal infection
  - Then mild proteinuria, mild to moderate hypertension
  - **Normal C3**
- Most important primary treatment is blood pressure control.

Alport Syndrome

The school nurse refers a 7-year-old boy because he failed his hearing test at school. The men in this patient's family have a history of renal problems, and a few of his maternal uncles are deaf. A urinalysis is obtained from the patient, which shows microscopic hematuria.

- Hereditary nephritis (X-linked dominant); renal biopsy shows **foam cells**
- Asymptomatic hematuria and intermittent gross hematuria **1–2 days after upper respiratory infection**
- **Hearing deficits (bilateral sensorineural, never congenital)** females have subclinical hearing loss
- **Ocular abnormalities (pathognomonic is extrusion of central part of lens into anterior chamber**

Henoch-Schönlein Purpura

- Small vessel vasculitis with good prognosis
- Present with purpuric rash, joint pain, abdominal pain
- Most resolve spontaneously; antiinflammatory medications, steroids
- See also rheumatic and vasculitic disorders chapter on this topic

Hemolytic Uremic Syndrome (HUS)

A 3-year-old child presents to the emergency center with history of bloody diarrhea and decreased urination. The mother states that the child's symptoms began 5 days ago after the family ate at a fast-food restaurant. At that time the patient developed fever, vomiting, abdominal pain, and diarrhea. On physical examination, the patient appears ill. He is pale and lethargic.

- **Most common cause of acute renal failure in young children**
- **Microangiopathic hemolytic anemia, thrombocytopenia, and uremia**
- Most from *E. coli* O157:H7 (shiga toxin–producing)
  - Most from undercooked meat or unpasteurized milk; spinach
  - Also from **Shigella, Salmonella, Campylobacter**, viruses, drugs, idiopathic
- Pathophysiology
  - Subendothelial and mesangial deposits of granular, amorphous material—vascular occlusion, glomerular sclerosis, cortical necrosis
  - Capillary and arteriolar endothelial injury → **localized clotting**
  - **Mechanical damage to RBCs as they pass through vessels**
  - **Intrarenal platelet adhesion and damage** (abnormal RBCs and platelets then removed by liver and spleen)
  - Prothrombotic state
- Clinical presentation
  - Most common <4 years old
  - Bloody **diarrhea**
  - **5–10 days after infection, sudden pallor, irritability, weakness, oliguria occur; mild renal insufficiency to acute renal failure (ARF)**
  - Labs—hemoglobin 5–9 mg/dL, **helmet cells, burr cells, fragmented cells,** moderate reticulocytosis, white blood cells up to 30,000/mm^3, Coombs negative, **platelets usually 20,000–100,000/mm^3,** low-grade microscopic hematuria and proteinuria
- Many complications, including seizures, infarcts, colitis, intussusception, perforation,, heart disease, death
- Treatment
  - Meticulous attention to fluids and electrolytes
  - Treat hypertension
  - Aggressive nutrition (total parenteral nutrition [TPN])
  - Early peritoneal dialysis
  - **No antibiotics if *E. coli* O157:H7 is suspected—treatment increases risk of developing HUS**
  - Plasmapheresis or fresh frozen plasma—may be beneficial in HUS **not** associated with diarrhea or with severe central nervous system involvement
- Prognosis—more than 90% survive acute stage; small number develop ESRD (end-stage renal disease)

POLYCYSTIC KIDNEY DISEASE

Autosomal-Recessive Type (Infantile)
- Both kidneys **greatly enlarged** with many cysts through cortex and medulla
- **Microcysts** → development of **progressive interstitial fibrosis and tubular atrophy** → **renal failure**
- Also **liver disease**—bile duct proliferation and ectasia with hepatic fibrosis

- Clinical presentation
  - Bilateral flank masses in neonate or early infancy
  - May **present with Potter sequence**
  - Hypertension, oliguria, acute renal failure
  - About half have liver disease in newborn period
- Diagnosis
  - **Bilateral flank masses in infant with pulmonary hypoplasia (if severe)**
  - Oliguria and hypertension in newborn with absence of renal disease in parents
  - Ultrasound–prenatal and postnatal (numerous small cysts throughout)
- Treatment and prognosis
  - Symptomatic
  - Now more than 80% with 10-year survival
  - End-stage renal failure in more than half
  - **Need dialysis and transplant**

Autosomal-Dominant Type (Adults)

- **Most common hereditary human kidney disease**
- Both kidneys enlarged with cortical and medullary cysts
- Most present in **fourth to fifth decade,** but may present in children and neonates
- Renal ultrasound shows bilateral **macrocysts**
- Also **systemic cysts**—liver, pancreas, spleen, ovaries; **intracranial (Berry) aneurysm** (rarely reported in children)
- Diagnosis—**presence of enlarged kidneys with bilateral macrocysts with affected first-degree relative**
- Treatment—**control of blood pressure** (disease progression correlates with degree of hypertension); presentation in older children with favorable prognosis

DISEASES PRESENTING WITH PROTEINURIA

Nephrotic Syndrome

A 3-year-old child presents to the physician with a chief complaint of puffy eyes. On physical examination, there is no erythema or evidence of trauma, insect bite, cellulitis conjunctival injection, or discharge.

- **Steroid-sensitive minimal change disease is the most common nephrotic syndrome seen in children.**
- Features
  - **Proteinuria (>40 mg/m^2/hour)**
  - **Hypoalbuminemia (<2.5 g/dL)**
  - **Edema**
  - **Hyperlipidemia (reactive to loss of protein)**

Minimal Change Disease

- Clinical presentation
  - **Most common between 2 and 6 years of age**
  - May follow minor infections
  - **Edema**—localized initially around eyes and lower extremities; anasarca with serosal fluid collections less common
  - Common—diarrhea, abdominal pain, anorexia
  - Uncommon—hypertension, gross hematuria
- Diagnosis
  - Urinalysis shows proteinuria (3–4 +)
  - Some with **microscopic hematuria**
  - 24-hour urine protein—**40 mg/m^2/hour in children but now preferred initial test is a spot urine for protein/creatinine ratio >2**
  - **Serum creatinine usually normal** but may be increased slightly
  - **Serum albumin <2.5 g/dL**
  - **Elevated serum cholesterol and triglycerides**
  - **C3 and C4 normal**
- Treatment
  - Mild—outpatient management; **if severe—hospitalize**
  - Start **prednisone** for 4–6 weeks, then taper 2–3 months without initial biopsy
  - **Consider biopsy with hematuria, hypertension, heart failure, or if no response after 8 weeks of prednisone (steroid resistant)**
  - Sodium restriction
  - If severe—fluid restriction, plus intravenous 25% albumin infusion, followed by diuretic to mobilize and eliminate interstitial fluid
  - Re-treat relapses (may become steroid-dependent or resistant); may use alternate agents (cyclophosphamide, cyclosporine, high-dose pulsed methylprednisolone); renal biopsy with evidence of steroid dependency
- Complications
  - **Infection is the major complication**; make sure immunized against *Pneumococcus* and *Varicella* and check PPD
  - **Most frequent is spontaneous bacterial peritonitis (*S. pneumoniae* most common)**
  - Increased risk of thromboembolism (increased prothrombotic factors and decreased fibrinolytic factors) but really with aggressive diuresis
- Prognosis
  - Majority of children have **repeated relapses; decrease in number with age**
  - Those with steroid resistance and who have focal segmental glomerulosclerosis have much poorer prognosis (progressive renal insufficiency).

MALE GENITOURINARY DISORDERS

Undescended Testes

- **Most common disorder of sexual differentiation in boys (more in preterm)**
- Testes should be descended by **4 months** of age or will remain undescended
- Usually in inguinal canal, but some are ectopic
- Prognosis
  - Treated: bilateral (50–65% remain fertile), unilateral (85% remain fertile)
  - Untreated or delay in treatment: increased risk for **malignancy** (**seminoma** most common)
- **Surgery (orchiopexy) at 9–15 months**

Note

Differentiate **undescended testes** from **retractile testes** (brisk cremasteric reflect age >1 [can manipulate into scrotum]).

Testicular Torsion

- **Most common cause of testicular pain age >12 years**
- Clinical presentation—**acute pain and swelling; tenderness to palpitation**
- Testicle in transverse lie and retracted, no cremateric reflex
- Diagnosis—Doppler color flow ultrasound (only to determine direction of torsion and to guide manual detorsion, if urologist decides this is warranted; also to confirm successful detorsion in a completely asymptomatic patient)
- Treatment—**emergent surgery** (scrotal orchiopexy); if within 6 hours and <360-degree rotation, >90% of testes survive

Torsion of Appendix Testes

- **Most common cause of testicular pain age 2–11 years**
- Clinical presentation
  - **Gradual onset**
  - 3–5 mm, tender, inflamed mass at **upper pole of testis**
  - Naturally resolves in 3–10 days (bed rest, analgesia)
- Diagnosis
  - Clinical—**blue dot** seen through scrotal skin
  - Ultrasound if concerned with testicular torsion
  - Scrotal exploration if diagnosis still uncertain

Epididymitis

- **Ascending, retrograde urethral infection → acute scrotal pain and swelling (rare before puberty)**
- **Main cause of acute painful scrotal swelling in a young, sexually active male**
- Urinalysis shows **pyuria** (can be *N. gonorrhoeae* [GC] or *Chlamydia*, but organisms mostly undetermined)
- Treatment—**bedrest and antibiotics**

Testicular Tumors

- 65% are malignant
- Palpable, hand mass that **does not** tranilluminate
- Usually **painless**
- Diagnosis
  - Ultrasound
  - Serum AFP, beta-HCG
- Treatment—radical orchiectomy

Endocrine Disorders

Learning Objectives

❏ Recognize and describe treatments for thyroid, parathyroid, and adrenal disorders

❏ Describe the epidemiology and treatment of childhood diabetes mellitus

. . . .

PITUITARY DISORDERS

Hypopituitarism

- **Deficiency of growth hormone ± other hormones; also delay in pubertal development is common; results in postnatal growth impairment corrected by growth hormone**
- Isolated growth-hormone deficiency or multiple pituitary deficiencies
  - Congenital—autosomal dominant, recessive, or X-linked recessive
  - Acquired—any lesion that damages the hypothalamus, pituitary stalk, or anterior pituitary (**most common is craniopharyngioma**)
- Clinical presentation
  - **Congenital** hypopituitarism:
    - **Normal size and weight at birth; then severe growth failure in first year**
    - Infants—**present with neonatal emergencies**, e.g., apnea, hypoglycemic seizures, hypothyroidism, hypoadrenalism in first weeks or boys with microphallus and small testes + cryptorchidism
    - Also have a variety of dysmorphic features; appearance
  - **Acquired** hypopituitarism:
    - Findings appear gradually and progress: growth failure; pubertal failure, amenorrhea; symptoms of both decreased thyroid and adrenal function; possible DI
    - If there is an **expanding tumor**: headache, vomiting; visual changes, decreased school performance; papilledema, cranial nerve palsies
- Laboratory evaluation
  - Screen for **low serum insulin-like growth factor (IGF)-1 and IGF-binding protein-3 (IGF-BP3)**
  - Definitive test—**growth-hormone stimulation test**
  - **Examine other pituitary function:**
    - Thyroid-stimulating hormone (TSH), T_4
    - Adrenocorticotropic hormone (ACTH), cortisol, dehydroepiandrosterone (DHEA) sulfate, gonadotropins, and gonadal steroids

Note

If there is a normal response to hypothalamic-releasing hormones, the pathology is located within the hypothalamus.

- Other studies
  - X-ray most helpful with **destructive lesions** (enlargement of sella, erosions)
  - Calcification
  - **Bone age—skeletal maturation markedly delayed (BA 75% of CA)**
  - **MRI is indicated in all patients with hypopituitarism.** (superior to CT scan)
- Differential diagnoses (the major ones)
  - **Systemic conditions** (Weight is often proportionally much less than height.)
  - **Constitutional delay** (delayed BA, delayed adolescent growth spurt, and pubertal development)
  - Familial **short stature** (BA = CA, short parents)
  - **Primary hypothyroidism**
  - **Emotional deprivation** (psychosocial dwarfism)
- Treatment
  - Classic growth-hormone deficiency—**recombinant growth hormone**
  - Need periodic thyroid evaluation—develop reversible hypothyroidism
- Indications—**growth hormone currently approved in United States for**
  - Documented growth-hormone deficiency
  - Turner syndrome
  - End-stage renal disease before transplant
  - Prader-Willi syndrome
  - Intrauterine growth retardation (IUGR) without catch-up growth by 2 years of age
  - Idiopathic pathologic short stature

Hyperpituitarism

- Primary—**rare; most are hormone-secreting adenomas**
- Majority are deficiencies of target organs and because of negative feedback, there are increases in hypothalamus and pituitary hormones
- Laboratory evaluation
  - Screen—**IGF-1 and IGF-BP3 for growth hormone excess;** confirm with a glucose suppression test
  - **Need MRI of pituitary**
  - **Chromosomes especially in tall males** (decreased upper- to lower-body segment ratio suggests XXY; mental retardation suggests fragile X)
  - **Thyroid tests**
- Management
  - Treatment only if prediction of adult height (based on BA) >3 SD above the mean or if there is evidence of severe psychosocial impairment
  - Trial of sex steroids (accelerates puberty and epiphyseal fusion)

Note

If the history suggests anything other than familial tall stature or obesity, or if there are positive physical findings, then the patient needs laboratory evaluation.

Prolactinoma

- Most common pituitary disorder of adolescents; more common in girls
- Headache, visual disturbances (with large tumors), galactorrhea, amenorrhea ± findings of hypopituitarism (again with large tumors)
- Diagnosis: increased serum prolactin level then best test, MRI
- Treatment: bromocriptine (still the only dopamine-agonist approved for children)

Physiologic Gynecomastia

- Breast tissue in the male: common (estrogen: androgen imbalance)
- Distinguish from pseudogynecomastia: adipose tissue in an overweight male
- May occur in newborns (estrogen effect) or adolescents (most common)
- Symmetric or asymmetric; may be tender
- Usually up to age 2 years
- If significant with psychological impairment, consider danzol (anti-estrogen) or surgery (rare)

Precocious Puberty

- Definition
  - Girls—sexual development age <8 years
  - Boys—sexual development age <9 years
- Most common etiologies
  - Sporadic and familial in girls
  - Hamartomas in boys
- Clinical presentation—advanced height, weight, and bone age; early epiphyseal closure and early/fast advancement of Tanner stages
- Evaluation
  - Screen—significant increase in leuteinizing hormone
  - Definitive—GnRH stimulation test; give intravenous GnRH analog for a brisk, leuteinizing hormone response
  - If positive, then order MRI
- Treatment—stop sexual advancement and maintain open epiphyses (stops BA advancement) with leuprolide

Incomplete Precocious Puberty

- Premature thelarche
  - Usually isolated, transient (from birth due to maternal estrogens)
  - May be first sign of true precocious puberty
- Premature adrenarche—early adrenal androgen production (variation of normal)—axillary, inguinal, and genital hair. It is familial.
- Premature menarche—very rare (other causes of bleeding much more common)

THYROID DISORDERS

Hypothyroidism

A 2-month-old patient appears to be having inadequate weight gain. His mother states he is constipated. On examination, he has decreased muscle tone, a large fontanel, a large tongue, and an umbilical hernia.

- *Congenital* hypothyroidism—**most are primary** (i.e., from thyroid gland)
  - Sporadic or familial; **with or without a goiter**
    - Most common is **thyroid dysgenesis** (hypoplasia, aplasia, ectopia); **no goiter**
    - Defect in **thyroid hormone synthesis—goitrous**; autosomal recessive
    - **Transplacental passage of maternal thyrotropin** (transient)
    - Exposure to maternal antithyroid drugs
    - Radioiodine exposure/fetal exposure to excessive iodine (topical iodine antiseptics) (now rare in U.S.)
    - Iodine deficiency or endemic goiter
    - Central hypopituitarism
  - Clinical presentation is known as "cretinism."
    - **Prolonged jaundice**
    - **Large tongue**
    - **Umbilical hernia**
    - **Edema**
    - **Mental retardation; developmental delay**
    - **Anterior and posterior fontanels wide**
    - **Mouth open**
    - **Hypotonia**
  - Other findings—weight and length normal at birth, feeding difficulties, apnea, sluggish, decreased appetite, increased sleep, constipation, decreased temperature, skin cold and mottled, peripheral anemia; apathetic appearance
  - Laboratory evaluation:
    - **Low serum T_4 or free T_4; increased TSH**
  - Treatment—**sodium thyroxine**
- *Acquired* hypothyroidism
  - **Hashimoto**; thryroiditis is most common cause; may be part of **autoimmune polyglandular syndrome**
  - Typically presents in **adolescence**
  - Other causes—iatrogenic (medications, irradiation, surgery, radioiodine); systemic disease (cystinosis, histiocytic infiltration)
- Clinical presentation
  - Many more girls than boys
  - **First sign usually deceleration of growth**

Note

Autoimmune Polyglandular Disease

Type I
- Hypoparathyroidism
- Addison disease
- Mucocutaneous candidiasis
- Small number with autoimmune thyroiditis

Type II *(Schmidt syndrome)*
- Addison disease, *plus:*
- Insulin-dependent DM
- With or without thyroiditis

- Then myxedema, constipation, cold intolerance, decreased energy, increased sleep, delayed osseous maturation, delayed puberty, headache, visual problems
- **Diffusely increased, firm, nontender thyroid;** but may be atrophic so can be non-goitrous
- Laboratory and treatment—same as congenital

Hyperthyroidism

A 12-year-old girl has a 6-month history of hyperactivity and declining school performance. Appetite is increased, but she shows no weight gain. Physical examination reveals a slight tremor of the fingers, mild exophthalmos, and a neck mass.

- Almost all cases are **Graves disease**
- **Peak at age 11–15 years;** girls > boys
- **Most with family history** of some form of autoimmune thyroid disease
- Findings
  - **Infiltration of thyroid and retro-orbital tissue** with lymphocytes and plasma cells → exopthalmos
  - **Lymphadenopathy and splenomegaly**
  - Thymic hyperplasia
- In whites, association with HLA-B8 and **DR3** is also seen with other DR3-related disorders (Addison disease, diabetes mellitus, myasthenia gravis, celiac disease).
- Clinical
  - Most signs and symptoms appear **gradually**
  - Earliest **usually emotional lability and motor hyperactivity**
  - **Decreased school performance**, tremor, increased appetite with weight loss, skin flushed with increased sweating, muscle weakness, **tachycardia, palpitations, arrhythmias, hypertension**
  - **Goiter, exophthalmos**
  - **Thyroid storm**—acute onset of hyperthermia, severe tachycardia, restlessness → rapid progression to delirium, coma, and death
- Laboratory evaluation
  - **Increased T_4, T_3, free T_4**
  - **Decreased TSH**
  - Measurable TRS-AB (and may have thyroid peroxidase antibodies)
- Treatment
  - **Propylthiouracil (PTU) or methimazole**
  - **Beta blockers** for acute symptoms (thyroid storm)
  - If medical treatment not adequate, radioablation or surgery; then treat as hypothyroid (daily thyroxine replacement)

Note

Thyroid cancer in children is uncommon, but you should know about medullary carcinoma (parafollicular cells), seen in 2 of the multiple endocrine neoplasias (MEN):

- **MEN IIA:** hyperplasia or cancer of thyroid *plus* adrenal medullary hyperplasia or pheochromocytoma *plus* parathyroid hyperplasia

- **MEN IIB (mucosal neuroma syndrome):** multiple neuromas *plus* medullary thyroid cancer *plus* pheochromocytoma

PARATHYROID DISORDERS

Hypoparathyroidism

- Parathyroid hormone (PTH) deficiency
- Etiologies
  - Aplasia/hypoplasia—most with **DiGeorge** or velocardiofacial syndrome
  - X-linked recessive—**defect in embryogenesis**
  - Autosomal dominant—mutation in calcium-sensing receptor
  - Postsurgical (thyroid)
  - Autoimmune—**polyglandular disease**
  - Idiopathic (cannot find other cause)
- Clinical presentation
  - Early—muscle pain/cramps, numbness, tingling
  - **Laryngeal and carpopedal spasm**
  - **Seizures (hypocalcemic seizures in newborn; think DiGeorge)**
- Laboratory evaluation
  - **Decreased serum calcium** (5–7 mg/dL)
  - **Increased serum phosphorus** (7–12 mg/dL)
  - Normal or low alkaline phosphatase
  - Low 1,25 $[OH]_2D_3$ (calcitriol)
  - Normal magnesium
  - **Low parathyroid hormone** (immunometric assay)
  - EKG: **prolongation of QT**
- Treatment
  - Emergency for neonatal tetany → intravenous 10% calcium gluconate and then 1,25$[OH]_2D_3$ (calcitriol); this normalizes the calcium
  - Chronic treatment with calcitriol or vitamin D_2 (less expensive) *plus* adequate calcium intake (daily elemental calcium)
  - Decrease foods high in phosphorus (milk, eggs, cheese)

Vitamin D Deficiency

- Most common cause of rickets
- Poor intake, inadequate cutaneous synthesis
- Low serum phosphate, normal to low serum calcium lead to increased PTH and increased alkaline phosphatase
- Increased 25-hydroxy vitamin D
- Fractures, rachitic rosary, craniotabe bone deformities
- Treatment: initial vitamin D replacement and calcium, then adequate dietary calcium and phosphate

Table 16-1. Lab Diagnosis of Parathyroid Disease

	PTH	Calcium	Phosphate	Alkaline Phosphatase
Primary Hypo	Decreased	Low	High	Normal
Pseudo Hypo	Increased	Low	High	NL or SL increased
Primary Hyper	Increased	High	Low	Increased
Secondary Hyper	Increased	NL to SL decreased	Low	Huge increase

ADRENAL DISORDERS

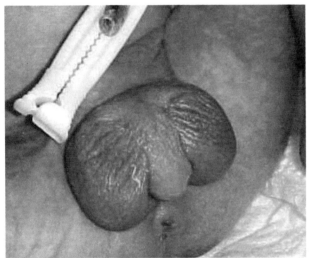

TheFetus.net.

Figure 16-1. Ambiguous Genitalia Seen in Congenital Adrenal Hyperplasia

Congenital Adrenal Hyperplasia (CAH)

A 1-month-old infant is seen with vomiting and severe dehydration. Physical examination reveals ambiguous genitalia; laboratory tests show hyponatremia.

- **21-Hydroxylase deficiency (most common)**
  - Autosomal-recessive enzyme deficiency
  - Decreased production of cortisol → **increased ACTH** –› **adrenal hyperplasia**
  - **Salt losing** (not in all cases; some may have normal mineralocorticoid synthesis)
  - Precursor steroids (17-OH progesterone) accumulate
  - **Shunting to androgen** synthesis → masculinizes external genitalia in females
  - Findings (with salt losing):
    ○ Progressive weight loss (through 2 weeks of age), anorexia, vomiting, dehydration
    ○ Weakness, hypotension

Note

Other 3 Main Defects in CAH

- **3-beta-hydroxysteroid deficiency:** salt-wasting, male and female pseudohermaphrodites, precocious pubarche; increased 17-OH pregnenolone and DHEA

- **11-beta-hydroxylase deficiency:** female pseudohermaphroditism, postnatal virilization, hypertension; increased compound S, DOC, serum androgens, and hypokalemia

- **17-alpha hydroxyl/17,20 lyase deficiency:** male pseudohermaphroditism, sexual infantilism, hypertension; increased DOC, 18-OH DOC, 18-OH corticosterone, and 17-alpha-hydroxylated steroids; hypokalemia

- Hypoglycemia, **hyponatremia**, hyperkalemia
  - **Affected females—masculinized external genitalia (internal organs normal)**
  - Males normal at birth; postnatal virilization
- Laboratory evaluation
  - **Increased 17-OH progesterone**
  - Low serum sodium and glucose, high potassium, acidosis
  - Low cortisol, increased androstenedione and testosterone
  - Increased plasma renin and **decreased aldosterone**
  - **Definitive test**—measure 17-OH progesterone before and after an intravenous bolus of ACTH
- Treatment
  - **Hydrocortisone**
  - **Fludrocortisone** if salt losing
  - **Increased doses of both hydrocortisone and fludrocortisone in times of stress**
  - Corrective surgery for females

Cushing Syndrome

- Exogenesis—most common reason is **prolonged exogenous glucocorticoid administration.**
- Endogenous
  - In infants—**adrenocortical tumor (malignant)**
  - Excess ACTH from **pituitary adenoma** results in **Cushing disease** (age >7 years)
- Clinical findings
  - **Moon facies**
  - **Truncal obesity**
  - **Impaired growth**
  - **Striae**
  - **Delayed puberty and amenorrhea**
  - **Hyperglycemia**
  - Hypertension common
  - Masculinization
  - **Osteoporosis with pathologic fractures**
- Laboratory evaluation
  - **Dexamethasone-suppression test (single best test)**
  - **Determine cause—CT scan (gets most adrenal tumors) and MRI (may not see if microadenoma)**
- Treatment—remove tumor; if no response, remove adrenals; other tumor-specific protocols

DIABETES MELLITUS

Type 1

An 8-year-old boy is seen in the emergency department with vomiting and abdominal pain of 2 days' duration. His mother states he has been drinking a lot of fluids for the past month, and reports weight loss during that time. Physical examination reveals a low-grade fever, and a moderately dehydrated boy who appears acutely ill. He is somnolent but asks for water. Respirations are rapid and deep. Laboratory tests reveal a metabolic acidosis and hyperglycemia.

- Etiology—T-cell–mediated autoimmune destruction of islet cell cytoplasm, insulin autoantibodies (IAA)
- Pathophysiology—low insulin **catabolic state**
  - Hyperglycemia → osmotic diuresis; when renal threshold for glucose reabsorption is reached (180 mg/dL) → glycosuria
  - Loss of fluid, electrolytes, calories, and dehydration
  - Accelerated lipolysis and impaired lipid synthesis → increased free fatty acids → ketone bodies → metabolic acidosis and Kussmaul respiration → decreased consciousness
- Clinical presentation
  - **Polyuria**
  - **Polydipsia**
  - **Polyphagia**
  - **Weight loss**
  - **Most initially present with diabetic ketoacidosis**
- Diagnostic criteria
  - Impaired glucose tolerance test
    - Fasting blood sugar 110–126 mg/dL or 2-hour glucose during OGTT<200 mg/dL but ≥125 mg/dL
  - Diabetes
    - Symptoms + random glucose ≥200 mg/dL or
    - Fasting blood sugar ≥126 mg/dL or
    - 2 hour OGTT glucose ≥200 mg/dL
  - **Diabetic ketoacidosis—hyperglycemia, ketonuria, increased anion gap, decreased HCO_3 (or total CO_2), decreased pH, increased serum osmolality**
- Treatment
  - Insulin administration, dosed primarily with meals
  - Testing before meals and at night
  - Diet modification
  - Close patient follow up

- Diabetic ketoacidosis:
  ○ **Insulin must be started at beginning of treatment.**
  ○ **Rehydration** also lowers glucose.
  ○ Monitor blood sugar, electrolytes; avoid rapid changes
  ○ Sodium falsely low
- Exercise
  ○ All forms of exercise or competitive sports should be encouraged.
  ○ Regular exercise improves glucose control.
  ○ May need additional CHO exchange

Type 2

- **Most common cause of insulin resistance is childhood obesity.**
- Symptoms more insidious
  - Usually excessive weight gain
  - Fatigue
  - Incidental glycosuria (polydipsia and polyuria uncommon)
- Risk factors
  - Age 10-19 years
  - Overweight to obese (BMI for age and sex >85%)
  - Non-Caucasian
  - History of type 2 DM in 1st- or 2nd-degree relatives
  - Having features of the metabolic syndrome
- Features of the Metabolic Syndrome
  - Glucose intolerance leads to L hyperglycemia
  - Insulin resistance
  - Obesity
  - Dyslipidemia
  - Hypertension
  - Acanthosis nigricans
- Screening and Treatment
  - **Who:** All who meet the BMI criteria + 2 risk factors
  - **How to screen:** fasting blood glucose every 2 years beginning at age 10 years or onset of puberty if above criteria are met
  - **Diagnosis:** same criteria (glucose levels) as adults
  - **Treatment:** first and most important is nutritional education and improved exercise level, but most will eventually need an oral hypoglycemic

Maturity-Onset Diabetes of Youth (MODY)

- Primary autosomal dominant defect in insulin secretion (6 types based on gene mutation)
- Diagnosis: 3 generations of DM with autosomal; dominant transmission and diagnosis of onset age <25 years
- Best test: molecular genetics for mutation (facilitates management and prognosis)

Orthopedic Disorders 17

Learning Objectives

❑ Recognize and describe treatments for childhood disorders of the hip, knee, foot, spine, and upper limbs

❑ Diagnose and describe treatments for osteomyelitis, septic arthritis, osteogenesis imperfecta, and bone tumors

DISORDERS OF THE HIP

Developmental Dysplasia of the Hip (DDH)

- General ligamental laxity
  - Family history
  - Significantly more females
  - Firstborn
  - Breech
  - Oligohydramnios
  - Multiple gestation
- Physical examination
  - **Barlow is most important examination**; will dislocate an unstable hip; is easily felt (clunk not a click)
  - **Ortolani**—reduces a recently dislocated hip (most at 1–2 months of age), but after 2 months, usually not possible because of soft-tissue contractions
- All infants with positive exams should **immediately be referred to an orthopedic surgeon** (per standard of practice of the AAP); no radiographic confirmation is needed
- If equivocal, can repeat exam in 2 weeks and if equivocal then **a dynamic U/S of the hips is the best test** (age <4 months) or hip x-ray (age >4 months)
- Treatment
  - Pavilk harness for 1–2 months
  - Surgery, casting
- Complications—acetabular dysplasia, leg length discrepancy

Legg-Calvé-Perthes Disease

A 5-year-old boy has developed progressive limping. At first painless, it now hurts to run and walk. The pain is in the anterior thigh. The pain is relieved by rest. Parents recall no trauma.

- **Idiopathic avascular necrosis** of the **capital femoral epiphysis** in immature, growing child
- More in males; 20% bilateral; sometimes after trauma
- Presentation—mild intermittent pain in anterior thigh with **painless limp** with restriction of motion
- Diagnosis—anterior/posterior and frog leg lateral x-ray shows compression, collapse, and deformity of femoral head
- Treatment
  - Containment (femoral head within acetabulum) with orthoses or casting
  - Bedrest
  - Abduction stretching exercises
  - If significant femoral deformity persists, surgical correction

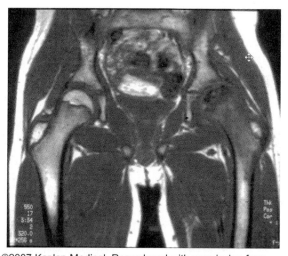

©2007 Kaplan Medical. Reproduced with permission from Dr. Philip Silberberg, University of California at San Diego

Figure 17-1. MRI Demonstrating Legg-Calve-Perthes Disease

Slipped Capital Femoral Epiphysis (SCFE)

- Most common adolescent hip disorder
- Either **obese** with delayed skeletal maturation, or **thin** with a **recent growth spurt**
- Can occur with an underlying endocrine disorder
- Clinical presentation
  - Pre-slip stable; exam normal; mild limp external rotation
  - Unstable slip; sudden-onset extreme pain; cannot stand or walk; 20% complain of knee pain with decreased hip rotation on examination

- Complications—osteonecrosis (avascular necrosis) and chondrolysis (degeneration of cartilage)
- Diagnosis—AP and frog-leg lateral x-ray, earliest finding: widening of physis without slippage (preslip); as slippage occurs, femoral neck rotates anteriorly while head remains in acetabulum
- Treatment—open or closed reduction (pinning)

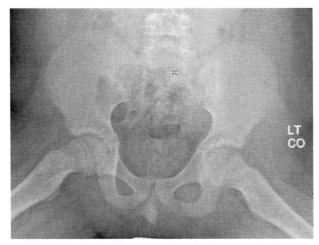

©2007 Kaplan Medical. Reproduced with permission from
Dr. Philip Silberberg, University of California at San Diego

Figure 17-2. X-ray of the Hips Demonstrating
Slipped Capitol Femoral Epiphysis

Transient Synovitis

- Viral; most 7–14 days after a nonspecific upper respiratory infection; most at 3–8 years of age
- Clinical presentation
  - Acute mild pain with **limp** and mild restriction of movement
  - Pain in groin, anterior thigh, and knee
- Diagnosis
  - Small effusion (±)
  - Slight increase in ESR
  - **Normal x-rays**
  - No to low-grade fever; non-toxic-appearing
- Treatment—bedrest and no weight-bearing until resolved (usually <1 week), then 1–2 weeks of limited activities

INTOEING

Metatarsus Adductus

- Most common in firstborn (deformation)
- Forefoot adducted from flexible to rigid
- Treatment—primarily nonsurgical; serial plaster casts before 8 months of age; orthoses, corrective shoes; if still significant in a child age >4 years, may need surgery

Talipes Equinovarus (Clubfoot)

A newborn is noted to have a foot that is stiff and slightly smaller than the other one. The affected foot is medially rotated and very stiff, with medial rotation of the heel.

- Congenital, positional deformation, or associated with neuromuscular disease
- Hindfoot equinus, hindfoot and midfoot varus, forefoot adduction (at talonavicular joint)
- Treatment
  - Complete correction should be achieved by 3 months (serial casting, splints, orthoses, corrective shoes); if not, then surgery

Internal Tibial Torsion

- **Most common cause of intoeing <2 years of age** (also because of in utero positioning); often with metatarsus adductus
- Measure prone thigh/foot angles
- No treatment needed—resolves with normal growth and development; takes 6–12 months (is physiologic)

Internal Femoral Torsion (Femoral Anteversion)

- Most common cause of intoeing ≥2 years of age; entire leg rotated inwardly at hip during gait
- Most are secondary to abnormal sitting habits (W-sitting).
- Treatment—observation; takes 1–3 years to resolve; surgery only if significant at >10 years of age

DISORDERS OF THE KNEE

Osgood-Schlatter Disease

- Traction apophysitis of tibial tubercle (**overuse injury**)
- Look for **active adolescent** (running, jumping)
- Swelling, tenderness, increased **prominence of tubercle**
- Treatment—**rest**, restriction of activities, knee immobilization, isometric exercises
- Complete resolution requires 12–24 months

Note

In **talipes equinovarus**, the patient's heel can't go flat on the exam surface (as opposed to metatarsus adductus, in which the heel can).

DISORDERS OF THE SPINE

Scoliosis

A 12-year-old girl is seen for routine physical examination. She voices no complaints. Examination is remarkable for asymmetry of the posterior chest wall on bending forward. One shoulder appears higher than the other when she stands up.

- **Most are idiopathic**; rarely, hemivertebra
- Others are congenital, with neuromuscular disorders, compensatory, or with intraspinal abnormalities.
- Slightly more females than males; more likely to progress in females
- Adolescent (>**11 years**) more common
- **Adams test bending forward at hips** —almost all with >**20-degree** curvature are identified in school screening programs (but many false positives)
- Diagnosis—x-ray is standard: posterior/anterior and lateral of entire spine gives greatest angle of curvature
- Treatment—trial brace for immature patients with curves 30–45 degrees and surgery for those >45 degrees (permanent internal fixation rods)

DISORDERS OF THE UPPER LIMB

Nursemaid Elbow

- When longitudinal traction causes radial head subluxation
- **History of sudden traction or pulling on arm**
- Physical exam reveals a child who refuses to bend his/her arm at the elbow
- Treatment—rotate hand and forearm to the supinated position with pressure of the radial head → reduction

OSTEOMYELITIS AND SEPTIC ARTHRITIS

- Etiology
  - **Osteomyelitis:**
    - *S. aureus* most common overall, in all
    - *Pseudomonas*—puncture wound
    - More *Salmonella* in sickle cell (*S. aureus* still most common)
  - **Septic arthritis:**
    - Almost all *S. aureus*
    - Most in young children; hematogenous; LE > UE and other parts of body
- Presentation
  - Pain with movement in infants
  - Older—fever, pain, edema, erythema, warmth, limp, or refusal to walk (acute, toxic, high fever)

Note

X-rays for patients with **osteomyelitis** are initially normal. Changes are not seen until 10–14 days.

- Diagnosis
  - Blood culture, CBC, ESR
  - Radiographic studies:
    - **Initial plain film** if diagnosis not obvious to exclude other causes—trauma, foreign body, tumor; trabecular long bones do not show changes for 7–14 days (septic arthritis shows widening of joint capsule and soft-tissue edema)
    - **Ultrasound for septic arthritis**—joint effusion, guide localization of drainage
    - **Best test is MRI for osteo**; very sensitive and specific
    - Bone scan—can be valuable to augment MRI, especially if multiple foci are suspected or vertebrate
  - Definitive—aspirate for culture and sensitivity
    - Osteomyelitis → bone biopsy for culture and sensitivity
    - Septic arthritis → ultrasound guided arthrocentesis for culture and sensitivity
- Treatment
  - Intravenous antibiotics—always cover for *Staphylococcus* initially (treatment for osteo much longer)

OSTEOGENESIS IMPERFECTA

- Susceptibility to fracture of long bones or vertebral compression from mild trauma
- **Most common genetic cause of osteoporosis;** all types caused by structural or quantitative defects in type I collagen
- **Autosomal dominant**
- **Clinical triad is fragile bones, blue sclera, and early deafness** (and short stature)
- Four types, from perinatally **lethal** to mild, nonlethal
- Diagnosis
  - May see fractures on prenatal ultrasound as early as 6 weeks
  - Rule out child abuse due to fracture and injury history.
  - Confirmed by collagen biochemical studies using fibroblasts cultured from a skin-punch biopsy
- Treatment—no cure; physical rehabilitation; fracture management and correction of deformities

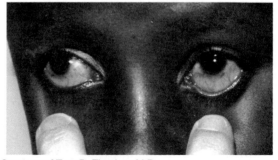
Courtesy of Tom D. Thacher, M.D.

Figure 17-3. Blue Sclera in Osteogenesis Imperfecta

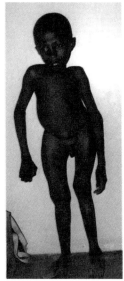

Courtesy of Tom D. Thacher, M.D.

Figure 17-4. Skeletal Malformation Due to Osteogenesis Imperfecta

BONE TUMORS

Table 17.1. Comparison of Osteogenic Sarcoma, Ewing Sarcoma, and Osteoid Ostcoma

	Osteogenic Sarcoma	Ewing Sarcoma	Osteoid Osteoma
Presentation	Second decade	Second decade	Second decade
M:F	Slightly greater in males	Slightly greater in males	3x greater in males
Predisposition	Retinoblastoma, radiation	None	Male gender
X-ray	Sclerotic destruction: **"sunburst"**	Lytic with laminar periosteal elevation: **"onion skin"**	Small round **central lucency** with sclerotic margin
Malignant	Yes	Yes	No
Metastases	Lungs, bone	Lungs, bone	N/A
Treatment	Chemotherapy, ablative surgery	Radiation and/or surgery	NSAIDs Surgery recommended when associated pain
Prognosis	70% cure without metastasis at diagnosis	60% cure without metastasis at diagnosis	Over time it may resolve spontaneously
Outcome if metastasis	≤20%	20–30%	N/A

Rheumatic and Vasculitic Disorders — 18

Learning Objectives

❏ Diagnose and describe management of juvenile idiopathic arthritis, systemic lupus erythematosus, Kawasaki disease, and Henoch-Schonlein Purpura

JUVENILE IDIOPATHIC ARTHRITIS (JIA)

A 7-year-old girl complains of pain and swelling of the left wrist and right knee off and on for the past 3 months. She has been previously healthy. The pain is worse in the morning and improves throughout the day. Physical examination is remarkable for swelling and effusion of the right knee, with decreased range of motion.

- Definition—idiopathic synovitis of peripheral joints associated with soft-tissue swelling and joint effusion
- Pathophysiology
  - Vascular endothelial hyperplasia and progressive erosion of articular cartilage and contiguous bone
  - Immunogenetic susceptibility and an external trigger
  - **DR8** and **DR5**
- Clinical presentation
  - **Morning stiffness**; easy fatigability
  - Joint pain later in the day, joint swelling, joints warm with decreased motion, and pain on motion, **but no redness**
- Criteria for diagnosis: the diagnosis of JRA is a clinical one, and one of exclusion. There are many diseases that mimic it and there are no pathognomonic diagnostic labs. The clinical exclusion of other diseases is essential, as lab studies may be normal.
  - Age of onset: <16 years
  - Arthritis in one or more joints
  - Duration: ≥6 weeks
  - Onset type by disease presentation in first 6 months

> **Note**
>
> A positive rheumatoid factor in JIA is indicative of a poor prognostic outcome.

- Exclusion of other forms of arthritis, other connective tissue diseases and vasculitides, **Lyme disease**, psoriatic arthritis, inflammatory bowel disease, **lymphoproliferative disease**

- Prognosis for severe and persistent disease
  - Young age at onset
  - RF+
  - Rheumatoid nodules
  - Persistence of anti-cyclic citrullinated peptide (CCP) antibodies (like RF, a marker for more severe disease)
  - Large number of affected joints
  - Involvement of hip, hands and wrists
  - Systemic onset JRA is the most difficult to control in terms of both articular inflammation and systemic manifestations (poorer with polyarthritis, fever >3 months and increased inflammatory markers for >6 months)

- Category of disease:
  - **Pauciarticular (oligoarthritis)**
    - **Pattern**: 1-4 joints affected in first 6 months; primarily knees (++) and ankles (+), less so the fingers; never presents with hip involvement
    - **Peak age** <6 years
    - **F:M** = 4:1
    - **% of all**: 50-60%
    - **Extra-articular**: 30% with anterior uveitis
    - **Labs**: ANA+ in 60%; other tests normal; may have mildly increased ESR, CRP
    - **Treatment**: NSAIDs + intraarticular steroids as needed; methotrexate occasionally needed
  - **Polyarticular, RF negative**
    - **Pattern**: 5 joints in first 6 months; both UE and LE small and large joints; may have C-spine and TMJ involvement
    - **Peak age**: 6-7 years
    - **F:M**: 3:1
    - **% of all**: 30%
    - **Extra-articular**: 10% with anterior uveitis
    - **Labs**: ANA+ in 40%; RF negative; ESR increased (may be significantly), but CRP increased slightly or normal; mild anemia
    - **Treatment**: NSAIDs + methotrexate; if not responsive, anti-TNF or other biologicals (as FDA-approved for children)
  - **Polyarticular RF positive**
    - **Pattern**: ≥5 joints as above but will be aggressive symmetric polyarthritis
    - **Peak age**: 9-12 years
    - **F:M**: 9:1
    - **% of all**: <10%
    - **Extra-articular**: rheumatoid nodules in 10% (more aggressive)

- Labs: RF positive; ESR greatly, CRP increased top normal; mild anemia; if anti-CCP antibodies are positive, then significantly worse disease

  - **Treatment**: long-term remission unlikely; early aggressive treatment is warranted

- **Systemic Onset**

  - **Pattern**: arthritis may affect any number of joints, but course is usually poly-articular, destructive and ultimately affecting hips, C-spine and TMJ

  - **Peak age**: 2-4 years

  - **F:M**: 1:1

  - **% of all**: <10%

  - **Extra-articular**: For initial diagnosis, in addition to arthritis in ≥1 joint, must have with or be preceded by **fever** ≥2 weeks documented to be quotidian (daily, rises to 39° then back to 37°) for at least 3 days of the ≥2-week period plus ≥1 of the following:

    ▸ **Evanescent** (nonfixed, migratory; lasts about 1 hour) erythematous, salmon-colored rash (linear or circular), most over the trunk and proximal extremities

    ▸ Generalized lymph node involvement

    ▸ Hepatomegaly, splenomegaly or both

    ▸ Serositis (pleuritis, pericarditis, peritonitis)

  - **Labs**: anemia, increased WBCs, increased ESR, CRP, increased platelets

  - **Treatment**: less responsive to standard treatment with methotrexate and anti-TNF agents; consider IL-1 receptor antagonists in resistant cases.

  - May have cervical spine involvement

- Labs

  - No best test

  - Increased acute-phase reactants; increased anemia of chronic disease

  - Increased **antinuclear antibodies (ANA) in 40–85%**, mostly with poly- and pauciarticular disease

  - **Positive rheumatoid factor (RF+)**—typically with onset of disease in an older child with polyarticular disease and development of rheumatoid nodules

- Treatment

  - Most with pauciarticular disease respond to **nonsteroidal antiinflammatory drugs (NSAIDs)** alone

  - Additional treatment—**methotrexate (safest and most efficacious of second-line agents)**; azathioprine or cyclophosphamide and biologicals

  - Corticosteroids (few indications):
    - Overwhelming inflammation
    - Systemic illness
    - Bridge treatment

  - Ophthalmology follow up; physical therapy (PT)/occupational therapy

Table 18-1. JRA Prognosis

Category	Serology	Major Problems	Outcome
Polyarticular disease	RF+	Older girls; hand and wrist; erosions, nodules, unremitting	Poor
	ANA+	Younger girls	Good
	Seronegative	—	Variable
Pauciarticular disease	ANA+	Younger girls; chronic iridocyclitis	Excellent, (except eyes)
	RF+	Polyarthritis, erosions, unremitting	Poor
	HLA B27	Older males	Good
	Seronegative	—	Good
Systemic	—	Pauciarticular	Good
	—	Polyarticular	Poor

SYSTEMIC LUPUS ERYTHEMATOSUS (SLE)

A 10-year-old girl presents with fever, fatigue, and joint pains. Physical examination is remarkable for a rash on the cheeks, swelling of the right knee, and pericardial friction rub. Initial laboratory tests reveal anemia and an elevated blood urea nitrogen and creatinine.

- Etiology
  - Autoantibodies, especially against nucleic acids including DNA and other nuclear antigens and ribosomes; blood cells and many tissue-specific antigens; immune complex deposition
    ◦ Immune complex deposition in the dermal/epidermal junction is **specific for SLE** (called the lupus band test)
    ◦ **Diffuse proliferative glomerulonephritis** significantly increases risk for severe renal morbidity (pathology varies from minimal mesangial changes to advanced sclerosing nephritis)
- Epidemiology
  - **90% female**
  - Compared with adults, children have **more severe disease and more widespread organ involvement**
  - Highest rate among African-Americans, Hispanics, Asians, Native-Americans and Pacific Islanders
  - Rare age <5 years and only up to 20% present age <16 years, so **usual presentation is mid-to-late adolescence**

Note

A pregnant woman with SLE will transfer IgG autoantibodies (usually anti-Ro) across the placenta at 12 to 16 weeks. This can cause a variety of manifestations, the most important being **congenital heart block**. All are temporary, except for the heart block, which may require permanent pacing.

- Clinical presentation
  - Most common is a **female with fever, fatigue, rash, hematological abnormalities (anemia of chronic disease or hemolytic; thrombocytopenia, leukopenia) and arthralgia/arthritis**
  - Renal disease is often asymptomatic, so need careful monitoring of UA and BP; presents as either flares with quiescent periods or a more smoldering disease (hypertension, glomerulonephritis, nephrosis, acute renal failure)
  - Neuropsychiatric complications can occur with or without active disease
  - Less common: lymphadenopathy, HSM/hepatitis, abdominal pain, diarrhea, melena
- Lab studies
  - **Nonspecific:** elevated ESR, CRP, platelets, anemia, elevated WBC or leukopenia/lymphopenia; decreased CH_{50}, C3, C4 (typically decreased in active disease and increases with treatment)
  - **+ANA:** present in 95-99% of SLE patients but has poor specificity; does not reflect disease activity; first screening test
  - **+anti-DS-DNA:** more specific (but not 100%) and may correlate with disease activity, especially nephritis
  - **+anti-Smith antibody (anti-Sm):** 100% specific but no disease activity correlation
  - **Antiribonucleoprotein antibodies:** increased with Raynaud's phenomenon (blanching of fingers) and pulmonary hypertension; high titer may be diagnostic of mixed CT disorder; antiribosomal-P-antibody is a marker for lupus cerebritis
  - **Anti-Ro antibody (anti-SSA):** IgG maternal antibodies crossing the placenta and produce transient neonatal lupus; may suggest Sjögren syndrome
  - **Anti-La (anti-SSB):** also increased risk of neonatal lupus; may be associated with cutaneous and pulmonary manifestations of SLE or isolated discoid lupus; also seen in Sjögren syndrome
  - **Antiphospholipid antibodies** (APL; including anticardiolipin): when a clotting event occurs in the presence of APL antibodies, the antiphospholipid syndrome is suspected:
    - Increased risk of arterial and venous thrombosis
    - Livedo reticularis
    - Raynaud's phenomenon produces cyanosis and then erythema, caused by cold stress or emotional stress; initial arterial vasoconstriction creates hypoperfusion then venous stasis, followed by reflex vasodilation
    - Positive lupus anticoagulant: may give a false-positive serological test for syphilis; also seen in patients with neurological complications
    - Recurrent fetal loss
  - Coombs positive: hemolytic anemia
  - Antiplatelet antibodies: thrombocytopenia
  - Antithyroid antibodies: autoimmune thyroiditis
  - Antihistone antibodies: may be found with **drug-induced lupus**; may act as a trigger in those prone to lupus or cause a reversible syndrome hepatitis is common (otherwise rare in children with lupus); more common drugs: minocycline, tetracycline, sulfasalazine, penicillin, nitrofurantoin, IH, many antihypertensives, anticonvulsants, procainamide, lithium, glyburide, statins, PTU, penicillamine, chlorpromazine, some biologicals

Note

Diagnosis of SLE—
"M.D. Soap 'n Hair"

- **M**alar rash
- **D**iscoid rash
- **S**erositis
- **O**ral ulcers
- **A**NA-positive
- **P**hotosensitivity
- **N**eurologic disorders
- **H**ematologic disorders
- **A**rthritis
- **I**mmune disorders (**LE [lupus erythematosus] prep test**, anti-DNA, Smith)
- **R**enal disorders

- General principles of treatment
  - Sunscreen and direct sun avoidance
  - Hydroxychloroquine for all, if tolerated
  - NSAIDs for joints
  - Corticosteroids for more severe disease, especially renal
  - Steroid-sparing immunosuppressives for severe disease (proliferative GN, continued vasculitis, pulmonary hemorrhage, severe persistent CNS disease)
  - LMW heparin is drug of choice for thrombosis, APL, lupus anticoagulant

NEONATAL LUPUS

- Passive transfer of IgG across placenta; most is maternal **anti-Ro and anti-La**
- Mostly presents at age 6 weeks with annular or macular rash affecting the face, especially periorbital area, trunk and scalp after exposure to any UV light; generally lasts 3-4 months
- At risk for future pregnancies; baby is at some risk for future autoantibody disease
- May manifest with any SLE finding, but all resolve unless there is **congenital heart block (can be detected in utero at 16 weeks); is permanent; if it is third degree, pacing is usually required.**

KAWASAKI DISEASE

An 18-month-old has had fever for 10 days. He now has conjunctival injection, a very red tongue and cracked lips, edema of the hands, and a truncal rash.

Note

The most serious sequelae of Kawasaki disease are cardiac-related.

- Etiology
  - Many factors point to an infective cause but no specific organism has been found
  - Genetic susceptibility: highest in **Asians** irrespective of location and in children and sibs of those with KD
  - KD-associated antigen in cytoplasmic inclusion bodies of ciliated bronchial epithelial cells, consistent with viral protein aggregates; suggests respiratory portal of entry
  - Seems to require an environmental trigger
- Epidemiology
  - Asians and Pacific Islanders at highest risk
  - 80% present at age **<5 years** (median is 2.5 years) but may occur in adolescence
  - Poor outcome predictors with respect to coronary artery disease: very young age, male, neutrophilia, decreased platelets, increased liver enzymes, decreased albumin, hyponatremia, increased CRP, prolonged fever
- Pathology
  - **Medium size vasculitis, especially coronary arteries**
  - Loss of structural integrity weakens the vessel wall and results in ectasia or saccular or fusiform aneurysms; thrombi may decrease flow with time and can become progressively fibrotic, leading to stenosis

Note

Any child suspected of having Kawasaki disease should have an echocardiogram.

- Diagnosis

  Absolute requirement: fever ≥5 days (≥101° F), unremitting and unresponsive; would last 1–2 weeks without treatment **plus any 4 of the following**:

  – **Eyes:** bilateral bulbar conjunctivitis, non-exudative

  – **Oral:** diffuse oral and pharyngeal erythema, strawberry tongue, cracked lips

  – **Extremities:** edema and erythema of palms and soles, hands and feet acutely; subacute (may have periungual desquamation of fingers and toes and may progress to entire hand)

  – **Rash:** polymorphic exanthema (maculopapular, erythema multiforme or scarlatiniform with accentuation in the groin); perineal desquamation common ion acute phase

  – **Cervical lymphadenopathy:** usually unilateral and >1.5 cm, nonsuppurative

Associated symptoms: GI (vomiting, diarrhea, pain); respiratory (interstitial infiltrates, effusions); significant irritability (likely secondary to aseptic meningitis); liver (mild hepatitis, hydrops of gallbladder); GU (sterile pyuria, urethritis, meatitis); joints (arthralgias/arthritis—small or large joints and may persist for several weeks)

- **Cardiac findings**

  – **Coronary aneurysms**: up to 25% without treatment in week 2-3; approximately 2–4% with early diagnosis and treatment; giant aneurysms (>8 mm) pose greatest threat for rupture, thrombosis, stenosis and MI; best detected by 2D echocardiogram

  – **Myocarditis**: in most in the acute phase; tachycardia out of proportion to the fever and decreased LV systolic function; occasional cardiogenic shock; pericarditis with small effusions. About 25% with mitral regurgitation, mild and improves over time; best detected by 2D echocardiogram plus EKG

  – Other arteries may have aneurysms (local pulsating mass)

- **Clinical phases**

  – **Acute febrile:** 1-2 weeks (or longer without treatment), diagnostic and associated findings and lab abnormalities; WBC increased (granulocytes), normocytic / normochromic anemia, normal platelets in first 1-2 weeks; ESR and CRP must be increased (usually significantly for the ESR); sterile pyuria, mild increase in liver enzymes and bilirubin; mild CNS pleocytosis. **Most important tests at admission** are **platelet count, ESR, EKG, and baseline 2D-echocardiogram**.

  – **Subacute:** next 2 weeks; acute symptoms resolving or resolved; extremity desquamation, significant increase in platelet count beyond upper limits of normal (rapid increase in weeks 2-3, often greater and a million); coronary aneurysm, if present, this is the time of highest risk of sudden death. **Follow platelets, ESR and obtain 2nd echocardiogram**.

  – **Convalescent:** next 2-4 weeks; when all clinical signs of disease have disappeared and continues until ESR normalizes; **follow platelet, ESR and if no evidence of aneurysm, obtain 3rd echocardiogram;** repeat echo and lipids at 1 year. If abnormalities were seen with previous echo, more frequent studies are needed, and cardiology follow-up and echocardiograms are tailored to their individual status.

- **Treatment**

  – **Acute:** (at admission): **(a)** IVIG over 10-12 hours (mechanism unknown but results in rapid defervescence and resolution of clinical symptoms in 85-90%);

Note

Kawasaki disease is one of the few instances in pediatrics for which you would use aspirin. (It is usually avoided because of the risk of developing Reye syndrome.)

the IVIG gives the large drop in incidence of aneurysms. If continued fever after 36 hours, then increased risk of aneurysm; give 2nd infusion. (**b**) oral high dose aspirin (anti-inflammatory dosing) until afebrile 48 hours

- ○ If winter, give heat-killed **influenza vaccine** if not yet received (**Reye syndrome**); cannot give varicella vaccine acutely (live, attenuated vaccine and concurrent IVIG would decrease its effectiveness, so must delay any MMR and varicella vaccine until 11 months post-IVIG.
  - – **Subacute (convalescent)**: change ASA to low dose (minimum dose for antithrombotic effects as a single daily dose until ESR has normalized at 6-8 weeks and then discontinue if echocardiogram is normal; if abnormalities, continue indefinitely

- **Complications and prognosis**
  - – Small solitary aneurysms: continue ASA indefinitely; giant or numerous aneurysms need individualized therapy, including thrombolytic
  - – Long-term follow-up with aneurysms: periodic echo and stress test and perhaps angiography; if giant, catheter intervention and percutaneous transluminal coronary artery ablation, direct atherectomy and stent placement (and even bypass surgery)
  - – Overall- 50% of aneurysms regress over 1-2 years but continue to have vessel wall anomalies; giant aneurysms are unlikely to resolve
  - – Vast majority have normal health
  - – Acute KD recurs in 1-3%
  - – Fatality rate <1%; all should maintain a heart-healthy diet with adequate exercise, no tobacco and should have intermittent lipid checks.

HENOCH-SCHÖNLEIN PURPURA (HSP)

A 5-year-old boy is seen with maculopapular lesions on the legs and buttocks. He complains of abdominal pain. He has recently recovered from a viral upper respiratory infection. Complete blood cell count, coagulation studies, and electrolytes are normal. Microscopic hematuria is present on urine analysis.

- **Most common vasculitis among children in United States**; leukocytoclastic vasculitis (vascular damage from nuclear debris of infiltrating neutrophils) + **IgA deposition** in small vessels (arterioles and venules) of **skin, joints, GI tract and kidney.**
- Worldwide distribution, all ethnic groups; slightly greater in males; almost all age 3-10 years; occurs mostly in fall, winter and spring, many after an URI
- Infectious trigger is suspected, mediated by IgA and IgA-immune complexes
- Genetic component suggested by occasional family clusters
- Skin biopsy shows vasculitis of dermal capillaries and postcapillary venules with infiltrates of neutrophils and monocytes; in all tissues, immunofluorescence shows IgA deposition in walls of small vessels and smaller amounts of C3, fibrin and IgM
- Clinical presentation:
  - – Nonspecific constitutional findings
  - – Rash: **palpable purpura**, start as pink macules and then become petechial and then purpuric or ecchymotic; usually symmetric and in gravity-dependent areas (legs

and back of arms) and pressure points (buttocks); lesions evolve in crops over 3-10 days and may recur up to 4 months. Usually there is some amount of subcutaneous edema

- **Arthralgia/arthritis:** oligoarticular, self-limited and in lower extremities; resolves in about 2 weeks, but may recur

- **GI: in up to 80%:** pain, vomiting, diarrhea, ileus, melena, **intussusception**, mesenteric ischemia or perforation (purpura in GI tract)

- **Renal: up to 50%:** hematuria, proteinuria, hypertension, nephritis, nephrosis, acute or chronic renal failure

- Neurological: due to hypertension or CNS vasculitis, possible intracranial hemorrhage, seizures, headaches and behavioral changes

- Less common: orchitis, carditis, inflammatory eye disease, testicular torsion and pulmonary hemorrhage

- American College of Rheumatology diagnosis: need **2 of the following**:

  (a) palpable purpura

  (b) age of onset <10 years

  (c) bowel angina = postprandial pain, bloody diarrhea

  (d) biopsy showing intramural granulocytes in small arterioles and venules

- **Labs (none are diagnostic):** increased WBCs, platelets, mild anemia, increased ESR, CRP; stool + for occult blood; increased serum IgA. Must assess and follow BP, UA, serum Cr; GI ultrasound: ball wall edema, rarely intussusception; skin and renal biopsies would be diagnostic but are rarely performed (only for severe or questionable cases)

- Treatment: supportive and **corticosteroids, but only with significant GI involvement or life-threatening complications (but steroids do not alter course alter overall prognosis nor prevent renal disease** (c) for chronic renal disease – azathioprine, cyclophosphamide, mycophenolate mofetil.

- Outcome: Most significant **acute complications** affecting morbidity and mortality = serious GI involvement; renal complications are **major long-term** and can develop up to 6 months after initial diagnosis, but rarely if initial UA and BP are normal. Monitor all patients x 6months with BP and UA. Overall prognosis is excellent; most have an acute, self-limited disease; about 30% have >1 recurrence, especially in 4-6 months, but with each relapse symptoms are less. If more severe at presentation, higher risk for relapses. 1-2% with chronic renal disease and 8% ESRD.

Hematology 19

Learning Objectives

❏ Categorize anemias into those caused by inadequate production, those caused by acquired production, and congenital anemias

❏ Describe the pathophysiology, diagnosis, and treatment of megaloblastic and hemolytic anemias

❏ Recognize and describe management of thalassemias and hemoglobin disorders

❏ Demonstrate understanding of coagulation disorders

ANEMIAS OF INADEQUATE PRODUCTION

Physiologic Anemia of Infancy

- Intrauterine hypoxia stimulates erythropoietin → ↑ RBCs (Hb, Hct)
- High F_iO_2 at birth downregulates erythropoietin
- **Progressive drop in Hb over first 2–3 months** until tissue oxygen needs are greater than delivery (typically 8–12 weeks in term infants, to Hb of 9–11 g/dL)
- **Exaggerated in preterm** infants and earlier; nadir at 3–6 weeks to Hb of 7–9 g/dL
- In term infants—no problems, **no treatment;** preterm infants usually need transfusions depending on degree of illness and gestational age

Iron-Deficiency Anemia

An 18-month-old child of Mediterranean origin presents to the physician for routine well-child care. The mother states that the child is a "picky" eater and prefers milk to solids. In fact, the mother states that the patient, who still drinks from a bottle, consumes 64 ounces of cow milk per day. The child appears pale. Hemoglobin is 6.5 g/dL and hemotocrit 20%. Mean corpuscular volume is 65 fL.

- Contributing factors/pathophysiology
  - Higher bioavailability of iron in breast milk versus cow milk or formula
  - **Introducing iron-rich foods is effective in prevention.**

- Infants with decreased dietary iron typically are **anemic at 9–24 months** of age.
  - Caused by consumption of large amounts of **cow milk** and foods not enriched with iron
  - Also creates abnormalities in mucosa of gastrointestinal tract → **leakage of blood,** further decrease in absorption
- **Adolescents** also susceptible → high requirements during growth spurt, dietary deficiencies, menstruation
- Clinical appearances—**pallor most common;** also irritability, lethargy, pagophagia, tachycardia, systolic murmurs; long-term with neurodevelopmental effects
- Laboratory findings
  - First decrease in bone marrow hemosiderin (iron tissue stores)
  - Then decrease in serum ferritin
  - Decrease in serum iron and transferrin saturation → increased total iron-binding capacity (TIBC)
  - Increased free erythrocyte protoporhyrin (FEP)
  - Microcytosis, hypochromia, poikilocytosis
  - Decreased MCV, mean corpuscular hemoglobin (MCH), increase RDW, nucleated RBCs, low reticulocytes
  - Bone marrow—no stainable iron
- Treatment
  - **Oral ferrous salts**
  - Limit milk, increase dietary iron
  - Within 72–96 hours—peripheral reticulocytosis and increase in Hb over 4–30 days
  - Continue iron for 8 weeks after blood values normalize; repletion of iron in 1–3 months after start of treatment

Lead Poisoning

- Blood lead level (BLL) **up to 5 μg/dL** is acceptable.
- Increased risks
  - Preschool age
  - Low socioeconomic status
  - **Older housing (before 1960)**
  - Urban dwellers
  - African American
  - Recent immigration from countries that use leaded gas and paint
- Clinical presentation
  - **Behavioral changes** (most common: hyperactivity in younger, aggression in older)
  - **Cognitive/developmental dysfunction**, especially long-term (also impaired growth)
  - **Gastrointestinal**—anorexia, pain, vomiting, **constipation** (starting at 20 μg/dL)
  - Central nervous system—**related to increased cerebral edema, intracranial pressure (ICP** [headache, change in mentation, lethargy, seizure, coma → death])
  - Gingival lead lines

- Diagnosis
  - Screening—targeted blood lead testing at **12 and 24 months** in high-risk
  - Confirmatory **venous sample—gold standard blood lead level**
  - Indirect assessments—**x-rays of long bones (dense lead lines);** radiopaque flecks in intestinal tract (recent ingestion)
  - Microcytic, hypochromic anemia
  - Increased FEP
  - Basophilic stippling of RBC
- **Treatment—chelation** *(see* **Table 19-1)**

Table 19-1. Treatment for Lead Poisoning

Lead Level (µg/dL)	Management
5–14	Evaluate source, provide education, repeat blood lead level in 3 months
15–19	Same *plus* health department referral, repeat BLL in 2 months
20–44	Same *plus* repeat blood lead level in 1 month
45–70	Same *plus* chelation: single drug, preferably dimercaptosuccinic acid (succimer, oral)
≥70	Immediate hospitalization *plus* 2-drug IV treatment: – ethylenediaminetetraacetic acid plus dimercaprol

CONGENITAL ANEMIAS

Congenital Pure Red-Cell Anemia (Blackfan-Diamond)

A 2-week-old on routine physical examination is noted to have pallor. The birth history was uncomplicated. The patient has been doing well according to the mother.

- **Increased RBC programmed cell death → profound anemia by 2–6 months**
- **Congenital anomalies**
  - **Short stature**
  - Craniofacial deformities
  - Defects of upper extremities; **triphalangeal thumbs**
- Labs
  - Macrocytosis
  - Increased HbF
  - **Increased RBC adenosine deaminase (ADA)**

- **Very low reticulocyte count**
- Increased serum iron
- **Marrow with significant decrease in RBC precursors**
- Treatment
  - **Corticosteroids**
  - **Transfusions and deferoxamine**
  - Splenectomy; mean survival 40 years without stem cell transplant
- Definitive—**stem cell transplant** from related histocompatible donor

Congenital Pancytopenia

A 2-year-old presents to the physician with aplastic anemia. The patient has microcephaly, microphthalmia, and absent radii and thumbs.

Note

Blackfan-Diamond

Triphalangeal thumbs

Pure RBC deficiency

Fanconi

Absent/hypoplastic thumbs

All cell lines depressed

- Most common is **Fanconi anemia**—spontaneous chromosomal breaks
- Age of onset from infancy to adult
- Physical abnormalities
  - Hyperpigmentation and café-au-lait spots
  - **Absent or hypoplastic thumbs**
  - **Short stature**
  - Many other organ defects
- Labs
  - Decreased RBCs, WBCs, and platelets
  - Increased HbF
  - **Bone-marrow hypoplasia**
- Diagnosis—bone-marrow aspiration and cytogenetic studies for chromosome breaks
- Complications—increased risk of **leukemia (AML) and other cancers**, organ complications, and bone-marrow failure consequences (infection, bleeding, severe anemia)
- Treatment
  - **Corticosteroids and androgens**
  - **Bone marrow transplant definitive**

ACQUIRED ANEMIAS

Transient Erythroblastopenia of Childhood (TEC)

- **Transient hypoplastic anemia between 6 months–3 years**
  - Transient **immune suppression** of erythropoiesis
  - Often after nonspecific viral infection (not parvovirus B19)
- Labs—decreased reticulocytes and bone-marrow precursors, normal MCV and HbF

- Recovery generally **within 1–2 months**
- Medication not helpful; may need one transfusion if symptomatic

Anemia of Chronic Disease and Renal Disease

- Mild decrease in RBC lifespan and relative failure of bone marrow to respond adequately
- Little or no increase in erythropoietin
- Labs
  - Hb typically 6–9 g/dL, **most normochromic and normocytic (but may be mildly microcytic and hypochromic)**
  - Reticulocytes normal or slightly decreased for degree of anemia
  - Iron low without increase in TIBC
  - Ferritin may be normal or slightly increased.
  - Marrow with normal cells and normal to decreased RBC precursors
- Treatment—control underlying problem, may need erythropoietin; rarely need transfusions

MEGALOBLASTIC ANEMIAS

Background

- RBCs at every stage are larger than normal; there is an asynchrony between nuclear and cytoplasmic maturation.
- **Ineffective erythropoiesis**
- Almost all are **folate or vitamin B$_{12}$ deficiency** from malnutrition; uncommon in United States in children; more likely to be seen in adult medicine.
- Macrocytosis; nucleated RBCs; **large, hypersegmented neutrophils**; low serum folate; iron and vitamin B$_{12}$ normal to decreased; marked increase in lactate dehydrogenase; hypercellular bone marrow with megaloblastic changes

Folic Acid Deficiency

- Sources of folic acid—green vegetables, fruits, animal organs
- Peaks at 4–7 months of age—irritability, failure to thrive, chronic diarrhea
- Cause—inadequate intake (pregnancy, **goat milk feeding,** growth in infancy, chronic hemolysis), decreased absorption or congenital defects of folate metabolism
- Differentiating feature—low serum folate
- Treatment—daily folate; transfuse only if severe and symptomatic

Vitamin B$_{12}$ (Cobalamin) Deficiency

- Only animal sources; produced by microorganisms (humans cannot synthesize)
- Sufficient stores in older children and adults for 3–5 years; but in **infants born to mothers with deficiency, will see signs in first 4–5 months**
- Inadequate production (extreme restriction [**vegans**]), lack of intrinsic factor (congenital pernicious anemia [rare], autosomal recessive; also juvenile pernicious anemia [rare] or gastric surgery), impaired absorption (terminal ileum disease/removal)

Note

Hypersegmented neutrophils have >5 lobes in a peripheral smear.

Note

If autoimmune pernicious anemia is suspected, remember the Schilling test and antiparietal cell antibodies.

- Clinical—weakness, fatigue, failure to thrive, irritability, pallor, **glossitis**, diarrhea, vomiting, jaundice, many **neurologic symptoms**
- Labs—normal serum folate and decreased vitamin B$_{12}$
- Treatment—parenteral B$_{12}$

Table 19-2. Comparison of Folic Acid Versus Vitamin B$_{12}$ Deficiencies

	Folic Acid Deficiency	**Vitamin B$_{12}$ (Cobalamin) Deficiency**
Food sources	Green vegetables, fruits, animals	Only from animals, produced by microorganisms
Presentation	Peaks at 4–7 months	Older children and adults with sufficient stores for 3–5 years Infants born to mothers: first signs 4–6 months
Causes	Goat milk feeding Chronic hemolysis Decreased absorption Congenital defects of folate metabolism	Inadequate production (vegans) Congenital or juvenile pernicious anemia (autosomal recessive, rare) Gastric surgery Terminal ileum disease
Findings	Low serum folate with normal to increased iron and vitamin B$_{12}$	Normal serum folate and decreased vitamin B$_{12}$
Treatment	Daily folate	Parenteral vitamin B$_{12}$

HEMOLYTIC ANEMIAS

Hereditary Spherocytosis and Elliptocytosis

- Most **autosomal dominant**
- Abnormal shape of RBC due to **spectrin deficiency** → **decreased deformability** → **early removal of cells by spleen**
- Clinical presentation
  - **Anemia and hyperbilirubinemia in newborn**
  - **Hypersplenism, biliary gallstones**
  - Susceptible to aplastic crisis (parvovirus B19)
- Labs
  - Increased reticulocytes
  - Increased bilirubin
  - Hb 6–10 mg/dL
  - Normal MCV; **increased mean cell Hb concentration (MCHC)**
  - **Smear—spherocytes or elliptocytes diagnostic**

- Diagnosis
  - Blood smear, family history, increased spleen size
  - Confirmation—**osmotic fragility test**
- Treatment—transfusions, splenectomy (after 5–6 years), folate

Enzyme Defects

Pyruvate kinase (glycolytic enzyme)
- Wide range of presentation
  - Some degree of pallor, jaundice, and splenomegaly
  - Increased reticulocytes, mild macrocytosis, polychromatophilia
- Diagnosis—**pyruvate kinase (PK) assay** (decreased activity)
- Treatment—exchange transfusion for significant jaundice in neonate; transfusions (rarely needed), splenectomy

Glucose-6-phosphate dehydrogenase (G6PD)

A 2-year-old boy presents to the physician's office for an ear check. Three weeks earlier, the child had an ear infection that was treated with trimethaprim-sulfamethoxazole. On physical examination the patient is noted to be extremely pale. Hemoglobin and hematocrit are 7.0 g/dL and 22%, respectively.

- Two syndromes
  - **Episodic hemolytic anemia** (most common)
  - Chronic nonspherocytic hemolytic anemia
- **X-linked;** a number of abnormal alleles
- Episodic common among **Mediterranean, Middle Eastern, African, and Asian** ethnic groups; wide range of expression varies among ethnic groups
- Within 24–48 hours after ingestion of an **oxidant (acetylsalicylic acid, sulfa drugs, antimalarials, fava beans) or infection and severe illness** → rapid drop in Hb, hemoglobinuria and jaundice (if severe)
- Acute drop in Hb, saturated haptoglobin → free Hb and hemoglobinuria, **Heinz bodies**, increased reticulocytes
- Diagnosis—**direct measurement of G6PD activity**
- Treatment—prevention (avoid oxidants); supportive for anemia

HEMOGLOBIN DISORDERS

Sickle Cell Anemia (Homozygous Sickle Cell or S-Beta Thalassemia)

A 6-month-old, African-American infant presents to the pediatrician with painful swollen hands and swollen feet.

- Occurs in endemic malarial areas
- Single base pair change (thymine for adenine) at the sixth codon of the beta gene (valine instead of glutamic acid)
- Clinical presentation
  - Newborn usually without symptoms; development of hemolytic anemia over **first 2–4 months (replacement of HbF)**; as early as age 6 months; some children have **functional asplenia; by age 5, all have functional asplenia**
  - First presentation usually **hand-foot syndrome (acute distal dactylitis)**—symmetric, painful swelling of hands and feet (ischemic necrosis of small bones)
  - **Acute painful crises:**
    - Younger—mostly **extremities**
    - With increasing age—**head, chest, back, abdomen**
    - Precipitated by **illness, fever, hypoxia, acidosis**, or without any factors (older)
  - More extensive **vaso-occlusive crises** → ischemic damage
    - Skin ulcers
    - Retinopathy
    - Avascular necrosis of hip and shoulder
    - Infarction of bone and marrow (increased risk of *Salmonella* osteomyelitis)
    - **Splenic autoinfarction**
    - Pulmonary—**acute chest syndrome** (along with sepsis, are most common causes of mortality)
    - **Stroke** (peak at 6–9 years of age)
    - **Priapism**, especially in adolescence
  - **Acute splenic sequestration** (peak age 6 mos to 3 yrs); can lead to rapid death
  - Altered splenic function → increased susceptibility to infection, especially with **encapsulated bacteria (S. pneumococcus, H. influenzae, N. meningitidis)**
  - **Aplastic crisis**—after infection **with parvovirus B19**; absence of reticulocytes during acute anemia
  - Cholelithiasis—symptomatic gallstones
  - Kidneys—decreased renal function (**proteinuria first sign**); UTIs, papillary necrosis
  - Labs
    - Increased reticulocytes
    - Mild to moderate anemia
    - Normal MCV
    - If severe anemia: smear for **target cells,** poikilocytes, hypochromasia, **sickle RBCs,** nucleated RBCs, **Howell-Jolly bodies** (lack of splenic function); bone marrow **markedly hyperplastic**
  - Diagnosis
    - Confirm diagnosis with **Hb electrophoresis (best test)**
    - **Newborn screen**; use Hb electrophoresis
    - **Prenatal diagnosis** for parents with trait
- Treatment—Prevent complications:
  - Immunize (pneumococcal regular *plus* **23-valent**, meningococcal)
  - Start **penicillin prophylaxis** at 2 months until age 5

Note

Patients without a functioning spleen are predisposed to infection with encapsulated organisms. Pneumococcal vaccines 13 (PCV13) and 23 (PPSV23) are necessary.

      ◦ Educate family (assessing illness, palpating spleen, etc.)

      ◦ Folate supplementation

– Aggressive antibiotic treatment of infections

– Pain control

– **Transfusions** as needed

– Monitor for risk of stroke with **transcranial Doppler**

– **Hydroxyurea**

– **Bone-marrow transplant in selected patients age <16 years**

THALASSEMIAS

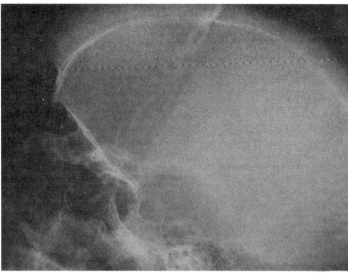

©2007 Kaplan Medical. Reproduced with permission from
Dr. Philip Silberberg, University of California at San Diego.

Figure 19-1. X-ray of Skull Demonstrating
"Hair on End" Appearance of Thallasemia

Alpha Thalassemia

- **Alpha thalassemia trait**: deletion of 2 genes

  – Common in African Americans and those of Mediterranean descent

  – Mild hypochromic, microcytic anemia (normal RDW) without clinical problems;

  – Often diagnosed as iron deficiency anemia; need molecular analysis for diagnosis

- **HgB H disease**: deletion of 3 genes; Hgb Barts >25% in newborn period and easily diagnosed with electrophoresis

  – At least one parent has alpha-thalassemia trait; later beta-tetramers develop (Hgb H—interact with RBC membrane to produce Heinz bodies) and can be identified electrophoretically; microcytosis and hypochromia with mild to moderate anemia; target cells present, mild splenomegaly, jaundice and cholelithiasis

  – Typically do not require transfusions or splenectomy; common in Southeast Asians

- **Alpha-thalassemia major**: deletion of 4 genes; severe fetal anemia resulting in hydrops fetalis
  - Newborn has predominantly Hgb Barts with small amounts of other fetal Hgb; immediate exchange transfusions are required for any possibility of survival; transfusion-dependent with only chance of cure (bone marrow transplant)

Beta Thalassemia Major (Cooley Anemia)

A 9-year-old has a greenish-brown complexion, maxillary hyperplasia, splenomegaly, and gallstones. Her Hb level is 5.0 g/dL and MCV is 65 mL.

- **Excess alpha globin chains** → **alpha tetramers** form; **increase in HbF** (no problem with gamma-chain production)
- Presents in second month of life with progressive **anemia, hypersplenism, and cardiac decompensation** (Hb <4 mg/dL)
- **Expanded medullary space** with increased expansion of **face and skull (hair-on-end)**; extramedullary hematopoiesis, **hepatosplenomegaly**
- Labs
  - Infants born **with HbF only** (seen on **Hgb electrophoresis**)
  - **Severe anemia**, low reticulocytes, increased nucleated RBCs, hyperbilirubinemia microcytosis
  - **No normal cells seen on smear**
  - **Bone-marrow hyperplasia; iron accumulates** → **increased serum ferritin and transferrin saturation**
- Treatment
  - Transfusions
  - **Deferoxamine** (assess iron overload with liver biopsy)
  - May need splenectomy
  - **Bone-marrow transplant** curative

HEMORRHAGIC DISORDERS

Evaluation of Bleeding Disorders

History provides the most useful information for bleeding disorders.

- **von Willebrand disease (vWD) or platelet dysfunction** → **mucous membrane bleeding, petechiae, small ecchymoses**
- **Clotting factors—deep bleeding with more extensive ecchymoses and hematoma**
- Laboratory studies
  - Obtain **platelets**, bleeding time, **PT, PTT**
    - If normal, von Willebrand factor (vWF) testing and thrombin time
    - If abnormal, further clotting factor workup
  - **Bleeding time**—platelet function and interaction with vessel walls; **qualitative platelet defects or vWD** (platelet function analyzer)

Note

Minor bleeds = von Willebrand

Deep bleeds = hemophilia

- Platelet count—thrombocytopenia is the most common acquired cause of bleeding disorders in children
- PTT—**intrinsic pathway:** from initiation of clotting at level of factor XII through the final clot (prolonged with factor VIII, IX, XI, XII deficiency)
- PT—measures **extrinsic pathway** after activation of clotting by thromboplastin in the presence of Ca^{2+}; **prolonged by deficiency of factors VII, XIII or anticoagulants**; standardized values using the **International Normalized Ratio (INR)**
- Thrombin time—measures the **final step: fibrinogen → fibrin**; if prolonged: **decreased fibrin or abnormal fibrin** or substances that interfere with fibrin polymerization (**heparin or fibrin split products**)
- Mixing studies: if there is a prolongation of PT, PTT, or thrombin time, then add normal plasma to the patient's and repeat labs
  - **Correction of lab prolongation suggests deficiency of clotting factor.**
  - **If not or only partially corrected, then it is due to an inhibitor (most common on inpatient basis is heparin).**
  - **If it becomes more prolonged with clinical bleeding, there is an antibody directed against a clotting factor (mostly factors VIII, IX, or XI).**
  - **If there is no clinical bleeding but both the PTT and mixing study are prolonged, consider lupus anticoagulant (predisposition to excessive clotting).**
- Clotting factor assays—each can be measured; severe deficiency of factors VIII or IX = <1% of normal; moderate = 1–5%; mild = >5%
- Platelet aggregation studies—if suspect a **qualitative platelet dysfunction, ristocetin**

Table 19-3. Clinical Findings in Coagulopathies

	Factor VIII	Factor IX	vWF
Platelet	Normal	Normal	Normal
PT	Normal	Normal	Normal
PTT	↑	↑	↑
Bleeding time	Normal	Normal	↑
Factor VIII	↓	Normal	Normal
Factor IX	Normal	↓	Normal
vWF	Normal	Normal	↓
Sex	Male	Male	Male/female
Treatment	Factor VIII, desmopressin	Factor IX	Fresh frozen plasma, cryotherapy, DDAVP

Hemophilia A (VIII) and B (IX)

- 85% are A and 15% B; no racial or ethnic predisposition
- **X-linked**
- Clot formation is delayed and not robust → **slowing of rate of clot formation**
  - With crawling and walking—**easy bruising**
  - Hallmark is **hemarthroses**—earliest in ankles; in older child, knees and elbows
  - Large-volume blood loss into iliopsoas muscle (inability to extend hip)—vague groin pain and hypovolemic shock
  - Vital structure bleeding—life-threatening
- Labs
  - 2× to 3× **increase in PTT** (all others normal)
  - **Correction with mixing studies**
  - Specific assay confirms:
    - Ratio of VIII:vWF sometimes used to diagnose carrier state
    - Normal platelets, PT, bleeding time, and vW Factor
- Treatment
  - Replace specific factor
  - **Prophylaxis now recommended** for young children with severe bleeding (intravenous via a central line every 2–3 days); prevents chronic joint disease
  - For mild bleed—patient's endogenous factor can be released with **desmopressin** (may use intranasal form)
  - Avoid antiplatelet and aspirin medications
  - DDAVP increases factor VIII levels in mild disease

Note

There is no way to clinically differentiate factors VIII and IX deficiencies. You must get specific factor levels.

von Willebrand Disease (vWD)

- Most common hereditary bleeding disorder; **autosomal dominant**, but more females affected
- Normal situation—vWF adheres to subendothelial matrix, and platelets then adhere to this and become activated; also **serves as carrier protein for factor VIII**
- Clinical presentation—**mucocutaneous bleeding** (excessive bruising, epistaxis, menorrhagia, postoperative bleeding)
- Labs—**increased bleeding time and PTT**
- **Quantitative assay for vWFAg, vWF activity** (ristocetin cofactor activity), plasma factor VIII, determination of vWF structure and platelet count
- Treatment—need to increase the level of vWF and factor VIII
  - Most with type 1 DDAVP **induces release of vWF**
  - For types 2 or 3 need replacement → **plasma-derived vWF-containing concentrates with factor VIII**

Other Bleeding Disorders

Vitamin K deficiency

- **Newborn needs intramuscular administration of vitamin K or develops bleeding diathesis**

- Postnatal deficiency—lack of oral intake, alteration in gut flora (long-term antibiotic use), malabsorption
- Vitamin K is fat soluble so deficiency associated with a decrease in factors **II, VII, IX, and X, and proteins C and S**
- Increased PT and PTT with normal platelet count and bleeding time

Liver disease

- **All clotting factors produced exclusively in the liver, except for factor VIII**
- Decreases proportional to extent of hepatocellular damage
- Treatment—**fresh frozen plasma** (supplies all clotting factors) and/or **cryoprecipitate** (supplies fibrinogen)

PLATELET DISORDERS

Immune Thrombocytopenic Purpura (ITP)

A 4-year-old child previously healthy presents with petechiae, purpura, and excessive bleeding after falling from his bicycle.

- **Autoantibodies** against platelet surface
- Clinical presentation
  - Typically 1–4 weeks after a nonspecific **viral infection**
  - Most 1–4 years of age → **sudden onset of petechiae and purpura with or without mucous membrane bleeding**
  - Most resolve within 6 months
  - **<1% with intracranial hemorrhage**
  - 10–20% develop chronic ITP
- Labs
  - **Platelets <20,000/mm^3**
  - **Platelet size normal to increased**
    Other cell lines normal
  - **Bone marrow—normal to increased megakaryocytes**
- Treatment
  - **Transfusion contraindicated** unless life-threatening bleeding (platelet antibodies will bind to transfused platelets as well)
  - No specific treatment if platelets >20,000 and no ongoing bleeding
  - If very low platelets, ongoing bleeding that is difficult to stop or life-threatening:
  - **Intravenous immunoglobulin for** 1–2 days
    ○ If inadequate response, then prednisone
  - Splenectomy reserved for older child with severe disease

Note

With ITP, the physical examination is otherwise normal; hepatosplenomegaly and lymphadenopathy should suggest another disease.

Oncology 20

Learning Objectives

❏ Categorize and describe management of leukemia and lymphomas

❏ Describe the epidemiology and management of brain tumors and other malignancies

LEUKEMIA AND LYMPHOMA

Acute Lymphoblastic Leukemia

A 5-year-old patient is brought to the physician's office with the chief complaint of a limp. The patient on physical examination has a low-grade fever, URI symptoms, hepatosplenomegaly, and petechiae.

Note

ALL is both CALLA (common acute lymphoblastic leukemia antigen) and TdT-positive.

- 77% of all childhood leukemias
- Onset brief and nonspecific (poor prognosis age <1 or >10 years at diagnosis)
  - Common—**bone and joint pain, especially lower extremities**
  - Then signs and symptoms of **bone marrow failure**—pallor, bruising, epistaxis, petechiae, purpura, mucous membrane bleeding, lymphadenopathy, hepato-splenomegaly, joint swelling
- Diagnosis
  - Peripheral blood:
    - ○ **Anemia**
    - ○ **Thrombocytopenia**
    - ○ **Leukemic cells not often seen early**
  - WBC mostly <10,000/mm^3 (atypical lymphocytes); poor prognosis if >100,000
  - **Best test is bone marrow aspirate → lymphoblasts**
  - If chromosomal abnormalities, poor prognosis
- Treatment
  - **Remission induction** (98% remission in 4–5 weeks; slow response = poor prognosis) with combination drugs
  - Second phase = **central nervous system (CNS) treatment**

- Intensive systemic *plus* intrathecal chemotherapy
  - **Maintenance phase** 2–3 years
- Complications
  - Majority is **relapse** (15–20%):
    - **Increased intracranial pressure (ICP) or isolated cranial nerve palsies**
    - **Testicular relapse** in 1–2% of boys
  - *Pneumocystis* pneumonia
  - Other infections because of immunosuppression
  - **Tumor lysis syndrome**—result of initial chemotherapy (cell lysis): hyperuricemia, hyperkalemia, hypophosphatemia → hypocalcemia (tetany, arrhythmias, renal calcinosis)
    - Treat with hydration and alkalinization of urine; prevent uric acid formation (allopurinol)
- Prognosis: >85% 5-year survival

Hodgkin Lymphoma

A 16-year-old boy presents with complaints of weight loss, fever, and night sweats. On physical examination, he is noted to have a nontender cervical lymph node that is 4–5 cm.

- Most in **15- to 19-year-olds**
- **Ebstein-Barr virus** may play a role; immunodeficiencies may predispose
- Diagnostic hallmark—**Reed-Sternberg cell** (large cell with multiple or multilobulated nuclei)
- Four major histologic subtypes
  - Lymphocytic predominant
  - Nodular sclerosing
  - Mixed cellularity
  - Lymphocyte depleted; now considered to be a high-grade non-Hodgkin lymphoma
- Clinical presentation depends on location
  - **Painless, firm cervical or supraclavicular nodes (most common presenting sign)**
  - **Anterior mediastinal mass**
  - Night sweats, fever, weight loss, lethargy, anorexia, pruritus
- Diagnosis
  - **Excisional biopsy of node (preferred)**
  - Staging from I to IV (single node or site to diffuse disease; multiple tests)
- Treatment
  - Determined by disease stage, large masses, hilar nodes
  - Chemotherapy
  - Radiation
- Prognosis—overall cure of 90% with early stages and >70% with more advanced

Non-Hodgkin Lymphoma

A 6-year-old boy presents to his primary care provider (PCP) with a nonproductive cough. A diagnosis of upper respiratory infection is made. However, the patient's symptoms persist, and he returns to his PCP. At this visit the patient is wheezing, and the PCP makes the diagnosis of reactive airway disease and prescribes an inhaled b2-agonist. The medication does not improve the symptoms; and the patient returns to the PCP for a third time. The patient is now complaining of cough and has a low-grade fever. The patient is diagnosed with clinical pneumonia; and an antibiotic is prescribed. Two days later the patient presents to the emergency department in respiratory distress. A chest roentgenogram shows a large mediastinal mass.

- Malignant proliferation of **lymphocytes of T-cell, B-cell, or intermediate-cell origin**
- **Epstein-Barr virus—major role in Burkitt lymphoma**
- Predisposition with congenital or acquired immunodeficiencies
- Three histologic subtypes
    - **Lymphoblastic** usually T cell, mostly **mediastinal masses**
    - **Small, noncleaved cell lymphoma**—B cell
    - **Large cell**—T cell, B cell, or indeterminate
- Presentation—depends on location
    - Anterior mediastinal mass (respiratory symptoms)
    - Abdominal pain, mass
    - Hematogenous spread
- Diagnosis—prompt because it is a very aggressive disease.
    - Biopsy
    - Any noninvasive tests to determine extent of disease: staging I to IV (localized to disseminated; CNS and/or bone marrow)
- Treatment
    - **Surgical excision of abdominal tumors**, chemotherapy, and monoclonal antibodies ± radiation
    - 90% cure rate for stages I and II

BRAIN TUMORS

Brain tumors are the second most frequent malignancy in children, with mortality 45%. They are more common age <7 years. Most are infratentorial (age 2–10 years, e.g., juvenile pilocytic astrocytoma, medulloblastoma); symptoms depend on the location.

The best initial test for all tumors is head CT scan. The best imaging test overall is MRI.

Some findings of brain tumors in general are severe persistent headaches, onset recurrent seizures, new onset neurologic abnormalities e.g., ataxia, behavioral/personality changes, deterioration of school performance, visual changes, III and VI nerve palsies, abnormal endocrine findings/new onset, papilledema.

Infratentorial Tumors

- **Most common**
- Low-grade, rarely invasive
- Most common—**juvenile pilocytic astrocytoma**
  - Classic site—**cerebellum**
  - Surgery, radiation, and/or chemotherapy
  - With complete resection, 80–100% survival

Others

- Malignant astrocytoma (includes glioblastoma multiforme)
- Medulloblastoma (midline cerebellar)
- Brain stem tumors (diffuse intrinsic with very poor outcome vs. low-grade gliomas)
- Ependymoma (most posterior fossa)

Supratentorial Tumors

Craniopharyngioma

A 14-year-old girl presents to the physician because of short stature. On physical examination, the patient is found to have bitemporal visual field defects. A head CT scan shows calcification at the sella turcica.

- **Most common**; 7–10% of all
- Minimal invasiveness; **calcification on x-ray**
- Major morbidity—**panhypopituitarism, growth failure, visual loss**
- Surgery and radiation; **no role for chemotherapy**

Optic nerve glioma

A 4-year-old boy with neurofibromatosis presents to the ophthalmologist with complaints of decreased visual acuity according to his parents. On physical examination, the patient has proptosis and papilledema.

- **Most frequent tumor of the optic nerve**; benign, slowly progressive
- **Unilateral visual loss, proptosis, eye deviation, optic atrophy, strabismus, nystagmus**
  - Increased incidence in **neurofibromatosis**
  - Treatment—observation:
    - If chiasm is involved—radiation/chemotherapy
    - Surgery if proptosis with visual loss

OTHER MALIGNANCIES

Wilms Tumor

A mother brings her 3-year-old child to the physician because she found an abdominal mass while bathing the child. The child has been in her usual state of health according to the mother. However, on review of the vital signs, the patient is noted to have an elevated blood pressure.

- **Nephroblastoma** (Wilm's tumor)
- **Second most common malignant abdominal tumor**
  - Usual age 2–5 years
  - One or both kidneys (bilateral in 7%)
  - **Associations:**
    - **Hemihypertrophy**
    - **Aniridia**
    - **Genitourinary anomalies**
    - **WAGR**
- Clinical presentation—most are **asymptomatic abdominal mass** (unless invasive at diagnosis, some with ↑ BP due to renal ischemia)
- Diagnosis
  - Best initial test–ultrasound
  - **Abdominal CT scan confirmatory test**
- Treatment
  - Surgery
  - Then chemotherapy and radiation
  - Bilateral renal—unilateral nephrectomy and partial contralateral nephrectomy
- Prognosis—54 to 97% have 4-year survival

Neuroblastoma

A 2-year-old child is brought to the physician because of bluish skin nodules, periorbital proptosis, and periorbital ecchymosis that have developed over the last few days. On physical examination, a hard smooth abdominal mass is palpated.

- **From neural crest cells, due to N-myc Oncogene; can occur at any site**
- 8% of childhood malignancies
- Most are
  - Adrenal
  - Retroperitoneal sympathetic ganglia
  - Cervical, thoracic, or pelvic ganglia
- Firm, palpable mass in flank or midline; **painful; with calcification and hemorrhage**
- Initial presentation often as **metastasis**—long bones and **skull, orbital**, bone marrow, lymph nodes, liver, skin

Note

Patients with neuroblastoma can present with ataxia or opsomyoclonus ("dancing eyes and dancing feet"). These patients may also have Horner syndrome.

- Diagnosis
  - Plain x-ray, CT scan, MRI (overall best)
  - Elevated urine **homovanillic acid (HVA)** and **vanillylmandelic acid (VMA)** in 95% of cases
  - Evaluate for spread—bone scan, bone marrow (neuroblasts) → staging from I (organ of origin) to IV (disseminated)
- Treatment
  - Surgery
  - Chemotherapy and radiation
  - Stem cell transplant (definitive)

Pheochromocytoma

- **Catecholamine-secreting** tumor from chromaffin cells
- **Most common site—adrenal medulla,** but can occur anywhere along abdominal sympathetic chain
- Children age 6–14 years; 20% are bilateral, and some with multiple tumors
- Autosomal dominant; associated with **neurofibromatosis,** *MEN-2A* and *MEN2B*, tuberous sclerosis, Sturge-Weber syndrome, and ataxia-telangiectasia
- Clinical presentation
  - **Episodic severe hypertension**, palpitations and diaphoresis, headache, abdominal pain, dizziness, pallor, vomiting, sweating, encephalopathy
  - Retinal examination—**papilledema, hemorrhages, exudate**
- Labs—significant increase in blood or **urinary levels of catecholamines and, metabolites**
- Diagnosis
  - Most tumors can be localized by **CT scan (best initial test)** and MRI, but extra-adrenal masses are more difficult.
  - Can use **I^{131} metaiodobenzylguanidine** (MBIG) scan → taken up by chromaffin tissue anywhere in body
- Treatment—**removal**, but high-risk
  - **Preoperative alpha and beta blockade** and fluid administration
  - Need prolonged follow up; may manifest later with new tumors

Note

Children with pheochromocytoma excrete predominantly norepinephrine-increased VMA and metanephrine. Children with neuroblastoma usually do not have hypertension, and major metabolites are dopamine and HVA.

Rhabdomyosarcoma

A mother brings her 3-year-old daughter to the physician for evaluation because the young girl has "grapes" growing out of her vagina.

- Almost any site, which determines presentation; determination of specific histologic type needed for assessment and prognosis
  - **Head and neck—40%**
  - **Genitourinary tract—20%**
  - **Extremities—20%**
  - Trunk—10%
  - Retroperitoneal and other—10%

- Increased frequency in **neurofibromatosis**
- Types
  - **Embryonal**—60%
    - Intermediate prognosis
  - **Botryoid** (projects; grapelike)—**vagina**, uterus, bladder, nasopharynx, middle ear
  - Alveolar—15%
    - Very poor prognosis
    - Trunk and extremities
  - Pleomorphic—adult form; very rare in children
- Clinical presentation
  - Mass that may or may not be painful
  - Displacement or destruction of normal tissue
  - Easily disseminates to lung and bone
- Diagnosis—depends on site of presentation
  - Biopsy, CT, MRI, U/S, bone scan
- Treatment—best prognosis with completely resected tumors (but most are not completely resectable)
  - Chemotherapy pre- and postoperatively; radiation

Neurology 21

Learning Objectives

❏ Describe the epidemiology and treatment of febrile and other seizure disorders

❏ Describe CNS anomalies, neurocutaneous syndromes, and neurodegenerative disorders

❏ Recognize and categorize encephalopathies

❏ Categorize and describe the epidemiology and genetics of neuromuscular disease

CENTRAL NERVOUS SYSTEM (CNS) ANOMALIES

Neural Tube Defects

Elevated **alpha-fetoprotein** is a marker for neural tube defects.

Spina bifida occulta

- Midline defect of vertebral bodies **without protrusion** of neural tissue; occasionally associated with other anomalies
- Most **asymptomatic and of no clinical consequence**
- May have **overlying midline lumbosacral defect** (patch of hair, lipoma, dermal sinus)

Tethered cord

- **Ropelike filum terminale persists and anchors the conus below L2**
- Abnormal tension—asymmetric lower extremity growth, deformities, bladder dysfunction, progressive scoliosis, diffuse pain, **motor delay**
- Most associated with a **midline skin lesion**
- **MRI needed for precise anatomy**
- Surgical transection

Meningocele

- Meninges herniate through defect in posterior vertebral arches
- **Fluctuant midline mass well covered with skin**; may transilluminate
- Must determine extent of neural involvement with MRI
  - CT scan of head for possible hydrocephalus
  - Surgery

Myelomeningocele

The pediatrician is called to the delivery room because an infant is born with a defect in the lumbosacral area.

- Strong evidence that **maternal periconceptional use of folate** reduces risk by half
- May occur anywhere along the neuraxis, but most are **lumbosacral**
- **Low sacral lesions—bowel and bladder incontinence and perineal anesthesia without motor impairment**

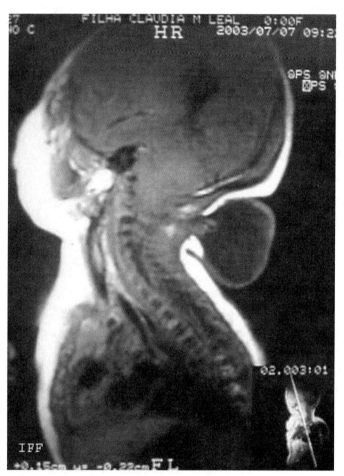

TheFetus.net

Figure 21-1. Arnold-Chiari Malformation, a Defect of the Hindbrain Usually Accompanied by Myelomeningocele

Note

Almost every child with a sacral or lower lumbar spine lesion will achieve some form of **functional ambulation**, and half of those with higher spine defects will have some degree of hip flexor and hip adductor movement.

- Midlumbar lesion—**saclike cystic structure** covered by thin, partially epithelized tissue
  - **Flaccid paralysis** below the level of the lesion is most common; no deep tendon reflexes (DTRs), no response to touch and pain
  - **Urinary dribbling, relaxed anal sphincter**
- 80% associated with **hydrocephalus; type II Chiari malformation**—may have symptoms of hindbrain dysfunction (feeding difficulty, choking, stridor, apnea, vocal cord paralysis, upper extremity spasticity)
- Evaluation and treatment
  - Must evaluate for other anomalies prior to surgery
  - Evaluate renal function
  - **Head CT scan for possible hydrocephalus**
  - Treatment—**ventriculoperitoneal shunt and correction of defect**

Hydrocephalus

A 2-month-old infant is noted to have a head circumference greater than the 95th percentile.

- Definition—**impaired circulation and absorption of CSF** or, rarely, from increased CSF production from a choroid plexus papilloma
- Types
  - **Obstructive** (noncommunicative) versus **nonobstructive** (communicative) from obliteration of subarachnoid cisterns or malfunction of arachnoid villi
    - Obstructive—most are **abnormalities of the cerebral aqueduct** (stenosis or gliosis; congenital, intrauterine infection, mumps, hemorrhage) **or lesions near the fourth ventricle** (brain tumor, Chiari malformation, Dandy-Walker malformation)
  - Nonobstructive—occurs mostly with **subarachnoid hemorrhage**; also with pneumococcal or TB meningitis or leukemic infiltrates
- Clinical presentation—depends on rate of rise of intracranial pressure
  - Infants:
    - **Increased head circumference**
    - **Bulging anterior fontanel**
    - Distended scalp veins
    - Broad forehead
    - **"Setting sun" sign**
    - Increased DTRs
    - Spasticity, clonus
  - Older child (subtler symptoms)
    - Irritability
    - Lethargy
    - Poor appetite

- o Vomiting
- o **Headache**
- o **Papilledema**
- o **Sixth-nerve palsy**
- Treatment for all types of hydrocephalus—shunting

Dandy-Walker malformation

- **Cystic expansion of fourth ventricle due to absence of roof**
- Associated **agenesis of posterior cerebellar vermis** and corpus callosum
- Presents with increasing head size and **prominent occiput,** long-tract signs, **cerebellar ataxia,** and delayed motor development, positive transillumination

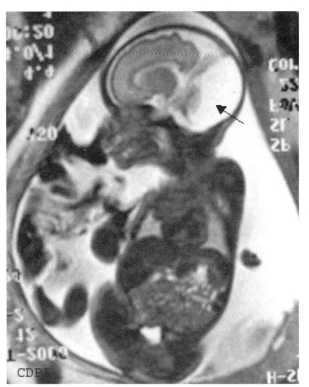

TheFetus.net

Figure 21-2. Dandy Walker Malformation, the Result of Agenesis or Hypoplasia of the Cerebellar Vermis, Cystic Dilatation of the Fourth Ventricle, and Enlargement of the Posterior Fossa

SEIZURES

Seizures are triggered recurrently from within the brain versus somatic disorders that may trigger a seizure from outside the brain. **Epilepsy** is present when **at least 2 unprovoked seizures occur >24 hours apart.**

Febrile seizures

An 18-month-old child is brought to the emergency center after having a generalized tonic-clonic seizure that lasted approximately 5 min. The parents say that the child had been previously well but developed cold symptoms earlier today with a temperature of 39°C (102°F).

- Occurs between age 6 months to 5 years; incidence peaks at age 14–18 months and may reoccur with fever
- Usually positive family history
- Temperature usually increases **rapidly** to >39°C (102°F)
- **Typical: generalized tonic-clonic seizures, <10–15 minutes; brief postictal period**
- **Atypical: >15 minutes, more than one in a day, and focal findings**
- Simple febrile seizure has **no increased risk of epilepsy**—risk for febrile seizures is increased with atypical seizure, family history of epilepsy, initial seizure before age 6 months, abnormal development, or preexisting neurologic disorder
    - Workup/Evaluation
        - Must determine cause of fever, must not look like meningitis
        - **No routine labs, no EEG, no neuroimaging**
    - Treatment—**control fever**

Partial Seizures

Simple

- **Asynchronous tonic or clonic movements; most of the face, neck, and extremities;** average duration 10–20 seconds
- Some have **an aura** and may verbalize during the attack; **no postictal period**
- EEG—**spike and sharp waves or multifocal spikes**
- Treatment—phenytoin and other anticonvulsants

Complex seizures

- **Impaired consciousness at some point,** may be very brief; one-third with aura (always indicates focal onset)
- **Automatisms** common after loss of consciousness (lip-smacking, chewing, swallowing, increased salivation)
- Interictal EEG—**anterior temporal lobe shows sharp waves or focal spikes**
- **MRI—many will show abnormalities in temporal lobe** (sclerosis, hamartoma, cyst, infarction, arteriovenous malformation [AVM], glioma)
- Treatment—**carbamazepine (drug of choice)** and other add-ons

Generalized Seizures

Absence (petit mal)

- **Sudden cessation of motor activity or speech with blank stare and flickering eyes**
- **More in girls; uncommon <5 years of age**
- **No aura**; usually <30 seconds; **no postictal period**
- EEG—**3/second spike and generalized wave discharge**
- Treatment—**ethosuximide (drug of choice)**, valproic acid (second line)

Tonic-clonic seizures

- May have **aura (focal onset; may indicate site of pathology)**; loss of consciousness, eyes roll back, tonic contraction, apnea
- **Then clonic rhythmic contractions** alternating with relaxation of all muscle groups
- Tongue-biting, loss of bladder control
- Semicomatose for up to 2 hours afterward with vomiting and bilateral frontal headache
- Treatment—**valproic acid, phenobarbital, phenytoin, carbamazepine**, and other add-ons

Myoclonic Seizures

- Repetitive seizures—**brief, symmetric muscle contraction** and loss of body tone with falling forward
- Five types, with variable severity, morbidity, and prognosis
- **Treatment—valproic acid** and others

Infantile Spasms

- **Symmetric contractions of neck, trunk, and extremities** (with extension episodes as well)
- Pathophysiology—increased corticotropin-releasing hormone (CRH): neuronal hyperexcitability
- Begin typically at 4–8 months of age
- Types
  - **Cryptogenic**—infant is normal prior to seizure with normal neurologic examination and development; **good prognosis**
  - **Symptomatic**—disease present prior to seizure (e.g., tuberous sclerosis); **poor control and mental retardation**
- EEG—**hypsarrhythmia** (asynchronous, chaotic bilateral spike-and-wave pattern)
- Treatment
  - **Adrenocorticotropic hormone (ACTH); drug of choice**
  - **Prednisone** and add-on of other anticonvulsants if no response

Note

Benign Myoclonus of Infancy

- Often confused with myoclonic seizures
- Clusters confined to the neck, trunk, and extremities
- EEG normal
- Good prognosis
- Goes away after 2 years; no treatment

Neonatal Seizures

- – Because of immaturity of CNS, **tend to have subtle seizures**; therefore, they are difficult to recognize
- Etiology
  - – **Hypoxic ischemic encephalopathy most common; seizure usually present within 12–24 hours after birth**
  - – CNS **infection**
  - – CNS **hemorrhage**
  - – **Structural** abnormalities
  - – Blood chemistry abnormalities
  - – **Inborn errors** of metabolism
  - – **Drug withdrawal**
  - – Evaluation:
    - ○ CBC; platelets
    - ○ Electrolytes, calcium, magnesium, phosphorus; glucose
    - ○ Lumbar puncture to exclude meningitis or bleed
    - ○ CT scan in term, ultrasound in preterm to diagnose bleed
    - ○ Blood and urine culture may be indicated (+CSF)
    - ○ Consider newborn screen for inborn errors of metabolism, if abnormal results suggestive or no diagnosis
    - ○ Treatment—lorazepam, phenobarbitol

Table 21-1. Neonatal Seizures

Cause	Presentation	Associations
Hypoxic ischemic encephalopathy	12–24 hours	Term; cerebral palsy
Intraventricular hemorrhage	1–7 days	Preterm
Metabolic	Variable	IODM (infant of diabetic mother), inborn errors of metabolism, DiGeorge syndrome
Infection	Variable	TORCH, maternal fever, sepsis/meningitis

NEUROCUTANEOUS SYNDROMES

A 6-year-old presents to the pediatrician for a routine evaluation. The child is noted to have 10 café-au-lait lesions as well as axillary freckling.

Neurofibromatosis (NF; von Recklinghausen Disease)

NF-1

- **Autosomal dominant**; but most with new mutation
- Every organ can be affected; features **present from birth but complications may be delayed into adulthood**
- Diagnosis—a good history and physical examination are needed to make the diagnosis.
  - **Two** of the following are needed:
    - At least 5 café-au-lait spots >5 mm prepubertal or at least 6 café-au-lait spots >15 mm postpubertal
    - Axillary/inguinal freckling
    - >2 iris Lisch nodules (seen on slit lamp only)
    - >2 neurofibromas or one plexiform neurofibroma
    - Osseous lesions, splenoid dysplasia or cortical thinning of long-bones (LE)
    - Optic gliomas
- Complications
  - CNS:
    - Low-grade **gliomas (optic), hamartomas**
    - **Malignant neoplasms** (astrocytoma, neurofibrosarcoma, and others)
    - Transient ischemic attack, hemiparesis, hemorrhage
    - Complex partial or generalized **seizures**
    - **Cognitive defects**, learning disabilities, attention deficit, speech abnormalities, psychiatric disturbances
  - **Renovascular hypertension or pheochromocytoma**
  - Increased incidence **of leukemia, rhabdomyosarcoma, Wilms tumor**
- Treatment
  - Genetic counseling
  - Early detection of treatable conditions
  - Annual ophthalmologic examination
  - Examine family members

NF-2

- Presentation
  - Primary feature—**bilateral acoustic neuromas**
  - Hearing loss
  - Facial weakness
  - Headache
  - Unsteady gait.
  - **Skin findings much less common** (glioma, meningioma, schwannoma)
  - CNS tumors common
- Treatment
  - Developmental and cognitive evaluation and diagnosis
  - Prevent pathological fractures if LE cortical thinning present

Tuberous Sclerosis

A 1-month-old infant presents with infantile spasms and has a hypsarrhythmic EEG pattern.

- **Autosomal dominant**; half with new mutations
- Wide range of manifestations within same family
- The younger the patient, the higher the likelihood of mental retardation
- Hallmark is CNS **tubers** found in **convolutions of cerebral hemispheres**; undergo calcification and project into ventricular cavity, causing obstruction of CSF flow and hydrocephalus.
- Clinical presentation
  - Infancy—with **infantile spasms** and characteristic skin lesions
    - **Ash-leaf macule**—hypopigmented; increased with Wood UV lamp
    - CT scan shows **calcified tubers** (but may not see till 3–4 years of age)
  - Childhood—**generalized seizures and skin lesions**
    - **Sebaceous adenoma**—red or clear nodules on nose and cheeks
    - **Shagreen patch**—rough, raised lesion with orange-peel consistency; most in lumbosacral area (midline)
- Diagnosis—**clinical:** characteristic skin lesions and seizure disorder
- Treatment—seizure control
- Complications
  - Retinal lesions—either mulberry tumor from optic nerve head or phakomas (round, flat, gray lesions in area of disc)–visual disturbances
  - Brain tumors much less common (but may see malignant astrocytoma)
  - Half have **rhabdomyoma of the heart** (can detect in fetus with echocardiogram); most spontaneously regress over first 2 years
  - **Renal lesion in most—either hamartoma or polycystic kidneys**
  - Pulmonary—cystic or fibrous changes

Sturge-Weber Syndrome (SW)

A newborn is examined in the nursery by the pediatrician. The patient is a product of a term spontaneous vaginal delivery without complications. On physical examination, the patient is noted to have a facial nevus.

- **Facial nevus (port wine stain), seizures, hemiparesis, intracranial calcifications, and mental retardation**
- **Nevus is always present at birth and always involves at least the upper face and eyelid**
- **Glaucoma** in ipsilateral eye
- Presentation
  - **Seizures in most** (focal tonic-clonic, **contralateral to the nevus**); becomes refractory and slowly develops **hemiparesis, mental retardation**
- Diagnosis
  - **Skull x-ray shows occipital-parietal calcifications (serpentine or railroad-track appearance) and intraocular pressure reading initially ($\uparrow$)**
  - **CT scan to highlight extent and show unilateral cortical atrophy and hydrocephalus ex vacuo**
- Treatment
  - Conservative if seizures are well controlled and development is not severely affected
  - Hemispherectomy or lobectomy—may prevent mental retardation and recalcitrant seizures if done in the first year of life
  - Regular intraocular pressure evaluation
  - Nevus—pulsed laser
  - Special education

ENCEPHALOPATHIES

Cerebral Palsy

- Group of motor syndromes from disorders of early brain development
  - Neurologic function may change or progress with time
  - Some have cognitive dysfunction
  - **Most born at term with uncomplicated labor and delivery**
    - Majority have no identifiable antenatal problems
    - **Only 10% with intrapartum asphyxia**
- **The most obvious manifestation is impaired ability of voluntary muscles (rigidity and spasticity).**
  - Other associations—seizures and abnormalities of speech, vision, and intellect
- Other risk factors—increased risk with intrapartum infection, **low birth weight,** (especially <1,000 g); most of these secondary **to intraventricular hemorrhage and periventricular leukomalacia**

- Diagnosis
  - MRI (location and extent of lesions or abnormalities)
  - If spinal involvement, MRI of spine
  - Hearing and visual evaluation
  - Genetic evaluation
  - Complete neurologic and developmental exams
- Treatment
  - Multidisciplinary team
  - Teach daily activities, exercises, assistance and adaptive equipment, surgical release procedures, communication equipment
  - Spasticity drugs (dantrolene, baclofen, botulinum toxin)
  - Psychological support

NEURODEGENERATIVE DISORDERS

Hallmark

- **Progressive deterioration of neurologic function**
  - Loss of speech, vision, hearing, and/or walking
  - Associated with seizures, feeding difficulties, and cognitive dysfunction
  - Regression of developmental milestones

Friedrich Ataxia

- Abnormal gene encoding for frataxin; autosomal recessive
- Onset of **ataxia** before <10 years of age
  - Slowly progressive
  - Loss of DTRs
  - Extensor plantar reflex
  - Weakness in hands and feet
  - Degeneration of posterior columns—loss of position and vibration sense
- **Explosive, dysarthric speech**
- Skeletal abnormalities, e.g., kyphoscoliosis
- **Hypertrophic cardiomyopathy—refractory congestive heart failure, death**

Wilson Disease

- Inborn error of **copper metabolism**; autosomal recessive
- Liver with or without CNS disease (neurologic, psychiatric)
- Liver symptoms first (any liver pathology), neurologic symptoms later (adolescent to adults)
  - Dystonia, tremors, basal ganglia problems
  - **Kayser-Fleischer rings**—pathognomonic (all will have with neuropsycho symptoms)

- MRI shows dilated ventricles with atrophy of cerebrum and lesions in thalamus and basal ganglia
- Diagnosis—**Suspect in any child with acute or chronic liver disease, unexplained neurologic disease, or behavioral or psychiatric changes**
    - **Best screen**—serum ceruloplasmin (decreased)
    - Confirm with liver biopsy—increased Cu content
    - Screen family members
- Treatment
    - Chelation with **penicillamine** (slows progression)
    - Definitive treatment with liver transplant

Sphingolipidoses

Tay-Sachs disease
- Deficient β-**hexosaminidase-A**, accumulate GM2
- Mostly in Ashkenazi Jews (carrier rate 1 in 30)
- Normal developmental until 6 months, then lag and lose milestones
- Seizures, hypotonia, blindness
- **Cherry-red macula**

Purine Metabolism Disorders

Lesch-Nyhan disease
- X-linked
- Purine metabolism disorder of purine metabolism → excess uric acid
- Delayed motor development after a few months
- **Self-mutilation and dystonia,** gouty arthritis, tophi, renal calculi
- Choreoathetosis, spasticity
- Diagnosis–**Analyze HPRT enzyme**
- Treatment
    - Manage renal complications, arthritis
    - Behavioral modification
    - Medication for reduction of anxiety and mood stabilization

NEUROMUSCULAR DISEASE

Spinal Muscle Atrophy (SMA)

A pediatrician examines an infant who is on the examination table in frog-leg position, with subdiaphragmatic retractions and absent tendon reflexes.

- **Degenerative disease of motor units beginning in the fetus and progressing into infancy; denervation of muscle and atrophy**
- Types
  - SMA 1 = **severe infantile (Werdnig-Hoffman disease)**
  - SMA 2 = late infancy, slower progression
  - SMA 3 = chronic juvenile (Kugelberg-Welander disease)
- Autosomal recessive
- Clinical presentation—SMA 1 presents in early infancy with
  - **Progressive hypotonia; generalized weakness;** Infant is flaccid, has little movement and poor head control
  - **Feeding difficulty**
  - **Respiratory insufficiency**
  - **Fasciculations of the tongue and fingers**
  - **Absent DTRs**
- Typically appear **brighter** than others of same age
- Diagnosis
  - **Simplest, most effective diagnosis is molecular genetic marker in blood for the *SMN* gene.**
  - EMG—fibrillation potential and other signs of denervation
  - Muscle biopsy shows a characteristic pattern of **perinatal denervation.**
- Treatment is supportive; there is no cure; most die in first 2 years of life

Myasthenia Gravis

A pediatrician examines an infant with poor sucking and swallowing since birth. The infant is noted to be a floppy baby with poor head control. There is associated ocular ptosis and weak muscles on repeated use.

- Immune-mediated neuronal blockade; motor end plate is less responsive due to, decreased number of available **acetylcholine receptors** secondary to **circulating receptor binding antibodies**; generally nonhereditary
- Clinical presentation
  - **Ptosis and extraocular muscle weakness is the earliest and most consistent finding.**
  - Dysphagia and facial weakness, and early infant feeding difficulties
  - Poor head control

Note

Transient Neonatal Myasthenia

- Neonates born to mothers with myasthenia; may have generalized hypotonia and weakness, feeding difficulties, and respiratory insufficiency from days to weeks

- May need ventilation and nasogastric feedings

- After antibodies wane, they are normal and have no risk for disease.

- Limb-girdle weakness and in distal muscles of hands
- **Rapid muscle fatigue**, especially late in the day
- May have respiratory muscle involvement
- Diagnosis
    - **EMG more diagnostic than muscle biopsy**—decremental response to repetitive nerve stimulation, reversed after giving cholinesterase inhibitor (edrophonium) → improvement within seconds
    - CPK is normal.
    - May have anti-acetylcholine (anti-ACh) antibodies (inconsistent)
- Treatment
    - Mild—many need no medication
    - Cholinesterase-inhibiting drugs—either neostigmine bromide PO or pyridostigmine
    - Severe—long-term prednisone; if no response, intravenous immunoglobulin (Ig), then plasmapheresis
    - Thymectomy—most effective if patient has high anti-ACh titers and symptoms for <2 years
- Complications—do not tolerate neuromuscular blockade and aminoglycosides potentiate

Hereditary Motor-Sensory Neuropathies (HMSNs)

HMSN I: Marie-Charcot-Tooth disease
- Progressive disease of peripheral nerves; **peroneal muscle atrophy; peroneal and tibial nerves**
- Autosomal dominant
- Clinical presentation
    - Asymptomatic until late childhood or adolescence but may have problem with gait as early as age 2 years
    - **Clumsy, fall easily; muscles of anterior compartment of lower leg become wasted → stork-like appearance**
    - **Pes cavus, foot drop**
    - **Claw hand** (in worse cases)
    - **Slowly progressive** through life, but normal lifespan and remain ambulatory
- Diagnosis
    - CPK is normal.
    - **Decreased nerve conduction velocities** (motor and sensory)
    - **Sural nerve biopsy** is diagnostic.
    - Blood molecular genetic diagnosis
- Treatment
    - **Stabilize ankles**
    - Surgical ankle fusion
    - Protection from trauma
    - If sensory problems, phenytoin or carbamazepine

Guillain-Barré Syndrome

- **Postinfectious polyneuropathy**—mostly motor; all ages; most with demyelinating neuropathy
- 10 days after a **nonspecific viral illness or *Campylobacter jejuni* or *Mycoplasma pneumoniae*—Landry ascending paralysis**
  - Symmetric proximal and distal muscles
  - Gradually over days to even weeks
  - May have **tenderness, pain, paresthesias early**
  - **Bulbar involvement** in half—dysphagia, facial weakness, **respiratory insufficiency**
  - May have **autonomic involvement**—blood pressure lability, bradycardia, asystole
  - Spontaneous recovery begins in 2–3 weeks; some have residual weakness; improvement in inverse direction
- Diagnosis
  - Significant **increase in CSF protein** with **normal glucose** and **no cells**
  - Reduced motor and sensory nerve conductions
- Treatment
  - Mostly supportive
  - **Admit all patients** (observe respiratory effort)
    - ◦ Mild-observation
  - **Intravenous immunoglobulin** 2–5 days
  - May need plasmapheresis, steroids, interferon, or other immunosuppressives

Muscular Dystrophy

Duchenne

A 3-year-old boy is brought to the pediatrician because he is very clumsy. According to his parents, he has difficulty climbing stairs and frequently falls. On physical examination hypertrophy of the calves is noted.

- Primary myopathy with genetic basis; is progressive and results in degeneration and death of muscle fibers; most common of the neuromuscular diseases in all races and ethnic groups; X-linked recessive
- Clinical presentation
  - First sign may be poor head control in infancy.
  - By year 2, may have subtle findings of hip-girdle weakness
  - **Gower sign** as early as age 3 years but fully developed by **age 5–6 years;** with hip-waddle gait and lordotic posturing
  - **Calf pseudohypertrophy** (fat and collagen) and wasting of thigh muscles
  - Most walk without orthotic devices until age 7–10 years, then with devices until 12; once wheelchair-bound, **significant acceleration of scoliosis**

- Progressive into second decade:
  - Respiratory insufficiency
  - Repeated pulmonary infections
  - Pharyngeal weakness (aspiration)
  - Contractures
  - **Scoliosis** (further pulmonary compromise)
  - **Cardiomyopathy** is a constant feature.
  - **Intellectual impairment** in all; IQ <70 in about 30%; most with **learning disabilities**

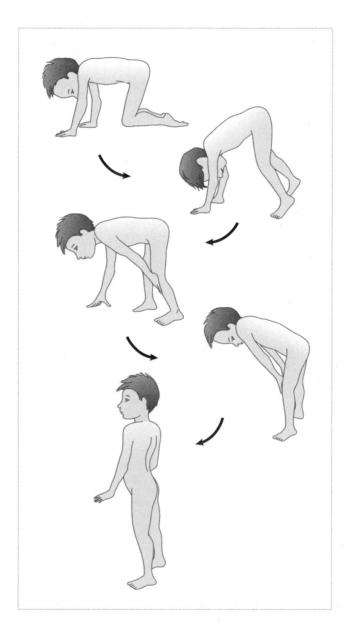

Figure 21-3. Gower Sign in Duchenne Muscular Dystrophy

- **Death usually around age 18 years** from respiratory failure in sleep, intractable heart failure, pneumonia, aspiration with obstruction

- Lab studies

    - **CPK—15,000–35,000** U/L (normal is <160 U/L) (initial screen for myopathy)

    - **Best initial test—molecular genetic diagnosis: deficiency or defective dystrophin cytoskeletal protein from gene at Xp21.2** (one-third will **not be diagnostic**)

    - **Muscle biopsy** to show the abnormal or absent dystrophin; most accurate test (do in the one-third who do not give a molecular diagnosis)

- Treatment—multidisciplinary team

    - **Digoxin** for heart failure (all patients need cardiology referral)

    - Vigorous treatment of pulmonary infections

    - Maintain good **nutrition**; good calcium supply (prevent osteoporosis)

    - **Physiotherapy**—delay contractions; **orthotic devices**, proper wheelchair, physiatrist

Myotonic Dystrophy

Myotonic dystrophy is the **second most common muscular dystrophy**.

- **Autosomal dominant** inheritance; CTG trinucleotide expansion at 19q13.3; causes multiple dysfunctions in multiple organ systems

- Involves both **striated and smooth muscle**

- Most common findings may be present at birth; the **severe congenital form** occurs in a baby born to a mother with symptomatic disease:

    - **Facial wasting: Inverted V-shaped upper lip, thin cheeks, scalloped concave temporalis muscles, narrow head, high arched palate**

    - **Hypotonia**: mild weakness and progressive wasting of DISTAL muscles especially hands, then dorsal forearm and anterior compartment of lower leg, then atrophy of proximal muscles

    - Progressive difficulty in climbing steps and lastly a Gower sign

    - **Slow progression** through childhood to adulthood but rare to lose ability to walk

    - NOTE: The distal distribution of muscle wasting is the exception to the general rule of myopathies having a proximal and neuropathies a distal distribution

    - **Myotonia**: not evident until age >5; very slow relaxation of muscle after a contraction, but NOT a painful muscle spasm (difficulty opening fist or relaxing grip)

- Other problems:

    - Poor speech articulation, slurred

    - Difficulty swallowing, aspiration pneumonia

    - Extraocular muscle weakness; cataracts

    - Slow GI emptying, constipation

    - Ineffective uterine contractions

    - Heart block and arrhythmia (not cardiomyopathy as in other dystrophies)

    - Many endocrine problems

        ○ Half with intellectual impairment

- Diagnosis: CPK as a screen (in the hundreds compared to MD); EMG classic myotonic findings; best test is DNA (blood); biopsy not needed

- Treatment: supportive

Learning Objectives

❏ Describe the presentation and emergency management of meningitis

❏ Describe the presentation and management of pertussis

❏ Recognize and describe treatment for mycobacteria, Lyme disease, and Rocky Mountain Spotted Fever

❏ Categorize and describe other important mycotic, viral, and helminthic diseases

MENINGITIS

A 6-year-old presents to the physician with the chief complaint of headache, vomiting, neck stiffness, and photophobia. Physical examination reveals an ill-appearing child unable to flex his neck without eliciting pain. Kernig and Brudzinski signs are positive.

Acute Bacterial (Older Than a Neonate)

- First 2 months of life (and some into month 3) represent maternal vaginal flora— group B *Streptococcus, E.coli, Listeria*
- Age 2 months to 12 years—*S. pneumoniae* (peaks in first 2 years), **N. meningitidis** (sporadic or in epidemics; direct contact from a daycare center or a colonized adult family member; increased in college freshmen living in dorms), and HiB (now **uncommon** due to many years of immunization)
- Pathology—meningeal inflammation and exudate
  - Most from hematogenous spread, initially from bacterial colonization of nasopharynx, and a prior or current viral infection may enhance pathogenicity
  - Rarely from an infection at a contiguous site (sinusitis, otitis media [OM], mastoiditis, orbital cellulitis)
- Clinical presentation
  - Several days of **fever, lethargy, irritability, anorexia, nausea, vomiting**
  - Then **meningeal irritation** (photophobia, neck and back pain, and rigidity)
    - ○ **Kernig sign:** flexing of hip 90° and subsequent pain with leg extension (inconsistent)

Note

Infants may not have positive Kernig or Brudzinski sign in meningitis but will have bulging fontanelles on physical examination.

- ° **Brudzinski sign:** involuntary flexing of knees and hips after passive flexing of the neck while supine (better test)
  - – Increased ICP suggested by headache, emesis, bulging anterior fontanelles, **oculomotor or abducens palsies**, hypertension with bradycardia, apnea, decorticate or decerebrate posturing, stupor, coma
- Diagnosis—**need lumbar puncture (LP) and blood culture in all** (90% have positive blood culture)
  - – **Contraindications to immediate LP**
    - ° Evidence of increased ICP
    - ° Severe cardiopulmonary problems requiring resuscitation
    - ° Infection of skin over site
    - ° Do not delay antibiotics for the CT scan.

Table 22-1. CSF Findings in Various Types of Meningitis

	Bacterial	Partially Treated	Granulomatous (TB)	Aseptic (Viral)
Cells/mL	200–5,000	200–5,000	100–500	100–700
Cytology	Polymorphonuclear neutrophil	Mostly polymorphonuclear neutrophil	Lymphocytes	Mostly lymphocytes
Glucose†	Low	Low	Low	Normal
Protein	High	High	High	Normal to slightly high
Gram stain	Positive	Variable	Negative	Negative
Culture	Positive	Variable	Positive	Negative
CIE or LA	Positive	Positive	Negative	Negative
Pressure	High	High	High	Normal

Definition of Abbreviations: CIE, counterimmunoelectrophoresis; LA, latex agglutination

†CSF glucose concentration should be considered in relation to blood glucose concentration; normally CSF glucose is 50–70% of blood glucose.

- Treatment

Table 22-2. Empiric Antibiotic Therapy Based on Age for Bacterial Meningitis

Age	Most Likely Organisms	Empiric Antibiotics
0-2 months	GBS, *E. coli*, L. monocytogenes	Ampicillin + cefotaxime
2-3 months	Above perinatal organisms + some *S. pneumoniae* + very little *H. influenza* type B	Ampicillin + cefotaxime/ ceftriaxone + vancomycin (assume resistant *S. pneumoniae*)
3 months – 2 years	*S. pneumoniae* + *N. meningitides*	Vancomycin + cefotaxime/ ceftriaxone
2-18 years	*N. meningitides* +	Vancomycin + cefotaxime/ ceftriaxone

Data support the use of IV dexamethasone added to the initial treatment of meningitis due to HiB, beginning with the first dose for 4 doses in children age >6 weeks (this will rarely be the case). Decreased incidence of fever, elevated CSF protein, and 8th cranial nerve damage.

- Complications
  - Increased ICP with herniation and seizures
  - Subdural effusion, especially in infants with HiB, can cause **seizures,** persistent fever; drain if symptomatic.
  - Cranial nerve palsies, stroke, thrombosis of dural venous sinuses
  - Most common sequelae is **hearing loss** (especially with pneumococcus)
  - Less common: mental retardation, developmental delay, visual impairment
- Prevention
  - **Chemoprophylaxis with rifampin for *N. meningitidis* and HiB, but not for *S. pneumoniae***
  - All close contacts regardless of age or immune status

Acute Meningococcemia

- Initially may mimic a viral disease (nonspecific)
- Any organ can be affected by **vasculitis and thromboembolic disease.**
- **Characteristic meningococcal rash** (black central arch and surrounding ring or erythema) often seen before more serious signs develop
- If fulminant—rapid progression: **septic shock, disseminated intravascular coagulation, acidosis, adrenal hemorrhage, renal and heart failure**
- Petechiae and purpura ± meningitis = **purpura fulminans (DIC)**
- Need high dose IV penicillin ASAP
- Chemoprophylaxis for close quarters (dorms, army barracks)

Viral (Aseptic) Meningitis

- Affects meninges and brain tissue variably; most are self-limited; person-to-person contact in summer and fall; most are enteroviruses
  - Arbovirus = arthropod-borne viruses; vectors are mosquitoes and ticks after biting infected birds or small animals; spreads to humans and other vertebrates
  - Rural exposure more common
  - Herpes simplex: **focal**; progresses to coma and death without treatment
  - Varicella zoster: most common presentation is cerebellar ataxia and acute encephalitis.
  - Cytomegalovirus: in immunocompromised, disseminated disease; or congenital infection but not in immunocompetent host
  - Epstein-Barr virus (EBV), mumps: mild but with 8th-nerve damage
- Clinical
  - **Headache and hyperesthesia in older children**
  - **Irritability and lethargy in infants**
  - **Fever, nausea, vomiting, photophobia, and neck, back, and leg pain**
  - Exanthems, especially **echovirus and coxsackie,** varicella, measles, and rubella
- Complications
  - Guillain-Barré syndrome, transverse myelitis, hemiplegia, cerebellar ataxia
  - Most completely resolve without problems except for the neonate with HSV (severe sequelae)
- Diagnosis
  - **PCR of CSF is the best test.**
  - Viral culture
- Treatment—supportive, except acyclovir indicated for herpes simplex virus (HSV)

PERTUSSIS

A 10-month-old child who is delayed in immunizations presents with a paroxysmal cough. The patient appears ill and continuously coughs throughout the examination. The patient has facial petechiae and conjunctival hemorrhages. In addition, the patient has post-tussive emesis.

- Cause—*Bordetella pertussis*
  - Endemic; very contagious; aerosol droplets
- Neither natural disease nor vaccination provides complete or lifelong immunity; **wanes after age 8–15 years**
  - Subclinical reinfection
  - Coughing **adolescents and adults are major reservoirs.**
- Clinical presentation of **whooping cough**
  - **Catarrhal phase** (2 weeks)—coldlike symptoms (rhinorrhea, conjunctival injection, cough)

- **Paroxysmal phase** (2–5 weeks)—increasing to severe coughing paroxysms, inspiratory "whoop" and facial petechiae; post-tussive emesis
    - **Convalescent phase** ≥ 2 weeks of gradual resolution of cough
- Diagnosis
    - **History may reveal incomplete immunizations**
    - **Gold standard is PCR of** nasopharyngeal aspirate 2–4 weeks after onset of cough, or a culture
- Treatment
    - **See immunization chapter**
    - **Supportive care**
    - **Always treat if suspected or confirmed: erythromycin for 14 days** (other macrolides with similar results) only decreases infectious period of patient; it *may* shorten the course of illness; also treat **all household members and any close contacts**

Bartonella (Cat-Scratch Disease)

A 6-year-old presents with a swollen 3×5-cm tender, erythematous, anterior cervical neck node. He denies a history of fever, weight loss, chills, night sweats, or sore throat. The patient's pets include a kitten, a turtle, and goldfish.

- Etiologic agent—*Bartonella henselae*
    - **Most common cause of lymphadenitis lasting >3 weeks**
    - Cutaneous inoculation (arthropod borne by cat flea); kittens transmit better than cats
    - Incubation period 3–30 days
- Clinical presentation
    - One or more 3- to 5-mm **red to white papules along the linear scratch** *plus* hallmark: **chronic regional lymphadenitis**
    - Other nonspecific findings: fever, malaise, headache, anorexia
    - Less common: abdominal pain, weight loss, hepatosplenomegaly, osteolytic lesion
    - Atypical presentation: Parinaud oculoglandular syndrome
- Diagnosis
    - **Clinical with history of scratch from cat**
    - Tissue: **PCR** and Warthin-Starry stain (shows gram-negative bacilli)
    - Serology: variable immunoglobulin IgG and IgM response (not good test)
- Treatment—**Antibiotics** not used as there is a discordance between in vitro and in vivo activity (use only for severe hospitalized cases) (usually self-limiting and resolves in 2–4 months); aspiration of large and painful lesions

Note

Parinaud oculoglandular syndrome consists of:

- unilateral conjunctivitis
- preauricular lymphadenopathy
- cervical lymphadenopathy
- occurs after rubbing the eye after touching a pet

MYCOBACTERIA

Tuberculosis

A 10-year-old child is referred by the school nurse because of a positive tuberculin skin test. The patient has been well, without any associated complaints.

- *M. tuberculosis*
- High-risk reservoirs—recent immigrants, low SES, HIV, elderly
- Primary complex—affects the **lung** with local infection with hilar adenopathy
- Latent infection—reactive TB skin test and absence of clinical or radiographic findings
- Diagnosis
  - Skin testing
    - Delayed hypersensitivity—Mantoux (PPD) test, (+) most often 4–8 weeks after inhalation
    - Positive reaction (**5, 10, 15** mm), depending on risk factors (*see* margin note)
  - Best—if can get sputum
    - **3 consecutive early A.M. gastric aspirates (still only 50%, even with PCR)**
    - A negative culture **never** excludes the diagnosis.
- Clinical Presentation
  - Primary TB usually asymptomatic in children; healthy host will wall off the organism; occasionally, low-grade fever, mild cough, malaise which resolve in 1 week
  - Infants more likely to have signs and symptoms
  - Reactivation rare, (esp. if acquired <2 years of age) occurs during adolescence
  - Small number with extrapulmonary presentation; symptoms depend on location
- Presentation
  - Primary pulmonary disease
    - Localized nonspecific infiltrate
    - Large adenopathy compared to infiltrate: compression → atelectasis and hyperinflation; most resolve completely
- Extrapulmonary
  - Erosion into blood or lymph = miliary
    - Lungs
    - Spleen
    - Liver
    - Bone and joints—Pott disease (destruction of vertebral bodies leading to kyphosis)
    - **TB meningitis**—mostly affects brainstem; CN III, VI, VII palsies and communicating hydrocephalus
  - If reactivation—fever, anorexia, malaise, weight loss, night sweats, productive cough, hemoptysis, chest pain

- Treatment
  - Latent TB
    - INH × 9 months
  - Primary pulmonary disease
    - INH + rifampin × 6 months, plus pyrazinamide in first 2 months
  - Increased community resistance
    - Add streptomycin, ethambutol or ethionamide
  - In some cases of meningitis, studies have shown decreased morbidity and mortality when **corticosteroids** added to regimen. Use adjunctively in patients with severe miliary disease and pericardial or pleural effusions.

Bacille Calmette-Guérin (BCG) Vaccination in the United States

- **Not routine**—variable efficacy, time-limited efficacy
- Only used in the following situations:
  - High-risk with close or long-term exposures
  - Continuous exposure to resistance strains
- Contraindicated in those with primary or secondary immune deficiencies

Perinatal Tuberculosis

- If mother has (+) PPD → obtain chest x-ray
- If chest x-ray (−) and clinically stable → no separation, no evaluation of baby, INH prophylaxis for mother for 9 months
- If mother has suspected TB at delivery → separate baby from mother until chest x-ray obtained
  - If mother has disease → treat infant with INH with no further separation from mother and treat mother with anti-TB therapy until mother is culture negative for 3 months

LYME DISEASE

A 6-year-old child presents with a rash after camping on Long Island with his family. On physical examination, the rash has a red raised border with central clearing.

Borrelia burgdorferi

- Most common vector-borne disease in the United States
- Most in southern New England, eastern Middle Atlantic states, and upper Midwest, with small endemic area along the Pacific coast
- *Ixodes scapularis*, i.e., the deer tick
- Clinical presentation: history of tick bite is helpful but absent in most; tick is small and often not seen by human eye; history of being in the woods or mountains should give suspicion

- Early disease
  - ○ **Local: erythema migrans** 3–32 days after bite at site of the bite; **target lesion (must be >10 cm in diameter)** often called "bulls-eye" rash; fever, headache, and malaise most common symptoms; without treatment, lesion resolves in 1–2 weeks
  - ○ **Early disseminated: secondary lesions**, smaller than the primary + constitutional symptoms + lymphadenopathy; uveitis and Bell palsy (may be only finding); carditis (myocarditis, heart block); CNS findings (neuropathy, aseptic meningitis)
  - Late disease: **arthritis** weeks to months later; affecting large joints, more likely to be chronic in adults
- Diagnosis
  - No definitive tests
  - Primarily **clinical and based on history + rash**
  - **Quantitative ELISA test and confirmatory Western blot if the ELISA is positive or equivocal**
- Treatment
  - Early
    - ○ **Doxycycline** 14–21 days (patients >8 years old); **amoxicillin** (patients age <8 years)
  - Ceftriaxone with meningitis or carditis (heart block)
  - Doxycycline or amoxicillin with Bell palsy
- Prognosis—excellent in children with permanent cure

ROCKY MOUNTAIN SPOTTED FEVER

A 17-year-old presents to the emergency department with his friends because of fever, headache, and a rose-colored rash that began on his ankles and is spreading. The patient and his friends have been camping in Virginia.

Rickettsia Rickettsii

- Consider in differential diagnosis of **fever, headache, and rash in summer months, especially after tick exposure**
- Seen now in every state; most in Southeast, especially in **North Carolina**
- Wooded areas, coastal grasses, and salt marshes
- Most April–September; most patients age <10 years
- Ticks are the natural hosts, reservoirs, and vectors (dog tick, wood tick, brown dog tick).
- Clinical presentation
  - Incubation period 2–14 days, then headache, fever, anorexia, myalgias, gastrointestinal (GI) symptoms early
  - After third day—**skin rash**
    - ○ Extremities first (palms, soles)
    - ○ Spreads rapidly
    - ○ Becomes petechial/hemorrhagic
    - ○ Palpable purpura

- Vascular obstruction, **due to vasculitis and thromboses, leads to gangrene**
- Hepatosplenomegaly
- CNS: delirium, coma, and other neurologic findings
- Myocarditis, acute renal failure, pneumonitis, shock
- Severe or fatal disease usually due to delay in diagnosis and treatment
- Diagnosis
  - **Strong clinical suspicion**
  - **Confirm with serologic tests;** fourfold increase in antibody titer (acute, convalescence)
- Treatment—**doxycycline or tetracycline in all patients regardless of age** (chloramphenicol in allergy only)

MYCOTIC INFECTIONS

Candida

A newborn infant is noted to have white plaques on his buccal mucosa that are difficult to scrape off with a tongue depressor. When removed, a small amount of bleeding is noted by the nurse. The infant just received a course of empiric antibiotics for suspected Group B β-hemolytic *Streptococcus* infection.

- Most human infections with *C. albicans;* part of normal gastrointestinal tract and vaginal flora of adults
- Oral infection = **thrush;** white plaques; seen with **recurrent or continuing antibiotic treatment and immunodeficiency and normally in breast-fed infants**
  - Diagnosis—**punctate bleeding with scraping**
  - Treatment—oral **nystatin;** if recalcitrant or recurrent, single-dose fluconazole

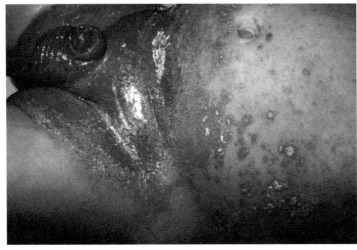

phil.cdc.gov

Figure 22-1. Diaper Rash Secondary to *Candida Albicans* Infection

- Diaper dermatitis: intertriginous areas of perineum; confluent, papular erythema with **satellite lesions**
  - Diagnosis—skin scrapings; see yeast with KOH prep, but not usually necessary in the presence of clinical findings
  - Treatment—**topical nystatin;** if significant inflammation, add 1% hydrocortisone for 1–2 days
- **Catheter-related fungemia** can affect any organ; may look like bacterial sepsis
  - Diagnosis—buffy coat, catheter tips, urine shows yeast, culture
  - Treatment—remove all catheters; **amphotericin B is drug of choice**
- Chronic mucocutaneous candidiasis—primary defect of T lymphocytes in response to *Candida*; often when **endocrine (diabetes mellitus) and autoimmune disease**

Cryptococcus Neoformans

- Soil contaminated with bird droppings, or in fruits and vegetables
- Predominant fungal infection in **HIV** patients; rare in children and immuno-competent
- Inhalation of spores; in immunocompromised (mostly in HIV patients) disseminated to **brain, meninges**, skin, eyes, and skeletal system; forms granulomas
- **Pneumonia most common presentation**; asymptomatic in many; otherwise, progressive pulmonary disease
- Diagnosis
  - **Latex agglutination—cryptococcal antigen in serum**; most useful for CSF infections
- Treatment
  - Oral fluconazole for 3–6 months if immunocompetent and only mild disease
  - Amphotericin B + flucytosine if otherwise
  - In HIV—lifelong prophylaxis with fluconazole

Coccidioidomycosis (San Joaquin Fever; Valley Fever)

A 14-year-old who lives in Arizona presents to the physician with a 10-day history of fever, headache, malaise, chest pain, and dry cough. He is currently in New York visiting relatives and is accompanied by his aunt. Physical examination reveals a maculopapular rash and tibial erythema nodosum.

- Inhaled arthroconidia from dust; no person-to-person spread
- Types
  - Primary (self-limiting)
  - Residual pulmonary lesions (transient cavity or chest x-ray)
  - Disseminating—can be fatal; more common in males, Filipino/Asians, blood group B
    - ○ Influenza-like symptoms
    - ○ Chest pain

- **Dry, nonproductive cough**
  - ○ Maculopapular rash
  - ○ **Tibial erythema nodosum**
- Diagnosis
  - Sputum should be obtained via bronchoalveolar lavage or gastric aspirates.
  - Diagnosis is confirmed by culture, **PCR**
- Treatment—most conservative; for those at high risk of severe disease, treatment as with histoplasmosis

Note

Disseminated Coccidiomycosis Triad
- Flu-like symptoms +/− chest pain
- Maculopapular rash
- Erythema nodosum

VIRAL INFECTIONS

Viral Exanthematous Disease

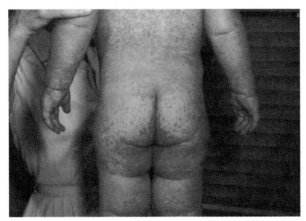

phil.cdc.gov.

Figure 22-2. Typical Appearance of Morbilliform Rash Seen in Measles Infection

Measles

A mother presents to the physician with her adopted daughter, who has just arrived in the United States from a foreign country. The immunization record is not up-to-date. The child has coryza, cough, conjunctivitis, and fever. The mother states that the child also has a rash that began cephalad and spread caudad. On physical examination, a morbilliform rash is seen over the body including the palms. Tiny grayish white dots are seen on the buccal mucosa next to the third molar.

- Rubeola—10-day measles
- RNA *Paramyxovirus*, **very contagious**
- Risk factors—Unimmunized entering high school or college
- Incubation—10–12 days before prodrome appears

- Prodrome—3 C's
  - Cough
  - Coryza
  - Conjunctivitis, then Koplik spots (grayish-white spots on buccal mucosa)
- Final—rash + fever (occur concurrently)
  - Rash—macular; starts at head (nape of neck and behind ears) and spreads downward; fades in same manner
- Diagnosis—mainly clinical
- Treatment—supportive, vitamin A (if deficient)
- Complications—otitis media (most common), pneumonia, encephalitis
- Prevention—immunization

Rubella

A 5-year-old child who has delayed immunizations presents with low-grade fever, a pinpoint rash, postoccipital and retroauricular lymphadenopathy, and rose spots on the soft palate.

- German, 3-day measles
- Risk factors/Etiology—Incubation 14–21 days; contagious 2 days before rash and 5–7 days after rash
- Clinical Presentation
  - Rash similar to measles, **begins on face** and spreads to rest of body, lasts approximately 3 days; concurrent with fever
  - **Retroauricular, posterior, and occipital lymphadenitis** are hallmarks.
  - Forscheimer spots—affect the soft palate and may appear before onset of the rash
  - Polyarthritis (hands) may occur in some patients, especially older females.
- Diagnosis—clinical
- Treatment—supportive
- Prevention—immunization with MMR vaccine
- Complications—congenital rubella syndrome seen if contracted during pregnancy (*see* Newborn chapter)

Roseola

A 15-month-old infant is brought to the physician because of a rash. The mother states that the patient had a fever of 40°C (104°F) for the last 3 days without any source of infection. She explains that the fever has resolved, but now the child has pink, slightly raised lesions on the trunk, upper extremities, face, and neck.

- Also known as exanthem subitum
- Etiology—febrile illness of viral etiology; due to infection with human herpes virus—HHV-6; peaks in children age <5 years, usually 6–15 months; incubation period 5–15 days
- Clinical Presentation
  - High fever (up to 41°C [106°F]) lasting a few days with only signs and symptoms of URI
  - By the 3rd or 4th day, the fever resolves and a maculopapular rash appears on the trunk, arms, neck, and face
    - Characteristic rose-colored rash begins as papules
- Diagnosis and treatment—clinical diagnosis based on age, history, and physical findings. No studies necessary and treatment is supportive.

Mumps

A 4-year-old child is brought to the clinic by his mother with a history of swelling in his face and fever for the last 4 days. His history includes incomplete immunizations due to religious beliefs. Physical examination reveals bilateral, tender facial swelling around the area of the masseter muscle and fever of 39.3°C (102.8°F).

- Etiology/Risk Factors—viral infection due to *Paramyxovirus* transmitted through airborne droplets and respiratory/oral secretions.,
  - Most common in winter/spring
  - Incubation period from 14–24 days
  - Contagious 1 day before and 3 days after swelling appears
  - History usually reveals inadequate or lacking immunizations
- Clinical Presentation
  - Constitutional findings: fever, headache, and malaise
  - Unilateral or bilateral salivary gland swelling, predominantly in the parotids
  - Orchitis (and oophoritis) possible, rare before puberty
    - May result in sterility only if **bilateral**
- Diagnosis—clinical and based upon history/physical findings
- Treatment—supportive
- Meningoencephalomyelitis most common complication; others include pancreatitis, thyroiditis, myocarditis, deafness, and dacryoadenitis

Varicella

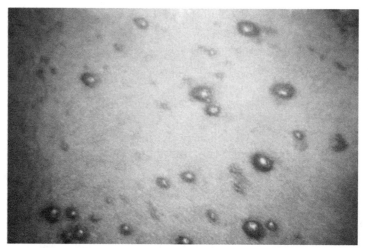

phil.cdc.gov

Figure 22-3. Chicken Pox is Characterized by Macules, Papules, Vesicles, and Crusts in Varying Stages of Healing

A 5-year-old child is brought to the emergency center because he has a temperature of 38.9°C (102°F) and is developing a pruritic rash. The rash appears to be in various stages of papules, vesicles, and crusts. It began on his trunk and spread to his extremities.

- Etiology/Risk Factors—due to varicella-zoster virus, a herpes virus
  - Incubation 10–21 days
  - Transmitted through respiratory secretions
  - Remains latent in sensory ganglia after recovery → reactivation in immunosuppressed
- Clinical Presentation—nonspecific symptoms and fever preceeding rash
  - **Pruritic rash in various stages**
    - **Macules → papules → vesicle → open vesicle → crust**
    - Lesions can turn hemorrhagic.
    - **Crops of lesions at same time**
- Clinical diagnosis—no labs
- Treatment
  - Supportive in immunocompetent; treat secondary infection
  - Consider acyclovir and VZIG in immunocomprised or those at risk for severe disease
- Complications—worse in adolescence (scarring)
  - Varicella pneumonia seen in 15–20%
  - Other sequelae include Guillian-Barré syndrome, encephalitis, cerebellar ataxia, postherpetic neuralgia, and Ramsay-Hunt syndrome.
  - Congenital varicella (*see* Newborn chapter)
- Prevention—second vaccine dose recommended

Erythema Infectiosum (Fifth Disease)

A 4-year-old is brought to the physician's office because she developed red cheeks that appear as if someone has slapped her, and a lacy rash on her upper extremities and trunk.

- Etiology—due to Parvovirus B19, a DNA virus; seen most commonly in spring
- Clinical Presentation
  - Mild systemic symptoms
  - Arthritis
  - Intensely red "slapped cheek" appearance
  - Lacy, reticular rash over trunk and extremities
  - Sparing of palms and soles
  - Rash may last up to 40 days
- Diagnosis—clinical; labs not routine **except** when diagnosing hydrops, then viral DNA in fetal blood is often helpful
- Complications—aplastic crisis in patients with hemolytic anemia; hydrops fetalis in neonates during materal infection in first trimester

Table 22-3. Common Childhood Infections with Exanthems

	Prodrome	Enanthem	Exanthem	Complications
Measles	• Cough • Coryza • Conjunctivitis • High fever	Koplik spots	Macules:, hairline, face, neck → trunk and extremities	• Otitis media • Pneumonia • Encephalitis • Subacute sclerosing panencephalitis
Rubella	Mild constitutional symptoms	Forscheimer spots	• Similar to measles • Posterior cervical & auricular nodes	Congenital rubella–teratogenic
Mumps	• Headache • Fever • Malaise • Muscle pain	Glandular swelling	Swollen parotid & submandibular glands	• Encephalitis • Orchitis • Pancreatitis
Varicella	• Low-grade fever • Malaise • URI symptoms	None	• Crops of papules, vesicles • Crusts at same time • Central to peripheral	• Superinfection • Zoster • Pneumonia • Hepatitis • Encephalitis • Congenital varicella
Fifth Disease	Mild URI symptoms	None	Slapped cheek → trunk → central clearing-lacey	Aplastic anemia
Roseola	• URI symptoms • Abrupt onset • High fever then breaks	None	Fever falls rapidly → fine macular rash on trunk and spreads to extremities	Febrile seizures
Scarlet Fever	Sore throat	• Exudative pharyngitis • Strawberry tongue	• Fine maculopapular rash (feels like sand paper, especially in antecubitus and inguinal areas) • Pastia lines	• Acute rheumatic fever • Glomerulonephritis

OTHER VIRAL DISEASES

Epstein-Barr Virus

A 22-year-old college student presents to the clinic complaining of fever, fatigue, and sore throat that have not improved for the last 2 weeks. Physical examination reveals generalized adenopathy most prominent in the anterior and posterior cervical nodes.

- Etiology/Risk Factors
  - **Infectious mononucleosis** (90%)
  - First human virus to be associated with **malignancy**
    - Nasopharyngeal carcinoma
    - **Burkitt lymphoma**
    - Others: Hodgkin disease, lymphoproliferative disorders, and leiomyosarcoma in immunodeficiency states
  - Transmitted in **oral secretions** by close contact (kissing disease); **intermittent shedding for life**
  - Incubation period: 30–50 days; most cases in infants and young children are clinically silent
- Clinical presentation
  - Insidious, vague onset: prodrome for 1–2 weeks with fever, fatigue, headache, myalgia, sore throat, abdominal pain
  - Generalized lymphadenopathy (most **in anterior and posterior cervical** and submandibular nodes; less often in axillary, inguinal, **epitrochlear** nodes), splenomegaly (half the cases; 2–3 cm), and a small number with hepatomegaly
  - Moderate to severe pharyngitis with tonsillar exudative enlargement
  - Small number with rashes (maculopapular); most will have rash if treated with **ampicillin or amoxicillin** (immune-mediated vasculitic rash)
- Diagnosis
  - **Atypical lymphocytosis**
  - **Heterophile antibodies (Monospot test)**
  - **IgM to viral capsid (Igm–VcA–EBV) antigen is the most valuable and specific (up to 4 months).**
- Treatment
  - Rest and symptomatic therapy
  - **No contact sports or strenuous activity with splenomegaly**
  - Short course of **steroids** for complications: incipient airway obstruction, thrombocytopenia with hemorrhage, autoimmune hemolytic anemia, seizures, meningitis
- Complications
  - **Splenic hemorrhage or rupture** (very rare); most in second week, most with trauma
  - Swelling of tonsils and oropharyngeal lymphoid tissue: **airway obstruction**
  - Neurological complications rare; Guillain-Barré syndrome
  - Aplastic anemia

Note

Infectious Mononucleosis Triad
- Fatigue
- Pharyngitis
- Generalized adenopathy

Note

Any exam question that mentions **onset of rash after** taking ampicillin or amoxicillin for URI-related symptoms, think mono first.

- Interstitial pneumonia
- Myocarditis
- Prognosis
  - Most cases resolve in 2–4 weeks; some disability that comes and goes for a few months is common; and there may be fatigue for a few years
  - There is no evidence of second attacks from EBV and no evidence that EBV is related to chronic fatigue syndrome

Influenza Viruses

A 14-year-old girl is brought to the physician's office by her mother. She has a 2-day history of fever of 39.7°C (103.5°F), headache, sore throat, refusal to eat, myalgia, chills and non-productive cough. Her current temperature in the clinic is 39.3°C (102.8°F).

- Etiology/Risk Factors
  - Three types—A, B, and C, with A and B being the primary pathogens of epidemic disease; now, also since 2009, H_1N_1
  - Migratory avian hosts may be responsible for spread.
  - Annual spread between Northern and Southern hemispheres; origin of new strains often traced to Asia
  - One or two predominant strains spread annually
  - Attack rate highest in the **young**; colder months in temperate climates
  - Transmission by small particle aerosol
- Clinical presentation
  - Predominantly respiratory illness
  - **Abrupt onset** with coryza, conjunctivitis, pharyngitis, and **dry cough**
  - Prominent systemic signs: **fever (2–4 days), myalgia, malaise, headache**
- Diagnosis
  - Virus can be isolated from nasopharynx early in course.
  - Rapid diagnostic test: **ELISA**
  - Can be confirmed serologically with acute and convalescent titers or PCR
- Treatment
  - Rest and adequate fluid intake
  - Control of fever
  - Antiviral drugs: decrease severity and duration if administered within first 48 hours of symptoms
- Complications—otitis media, pneumonia; secondary bacterial infection, myocarditis

Coxsackievirus

A 2-year-old infant is brought to the clinic with a vesicular rash in his mouth and on his palms and soles. Examination reveals a rash on his buttocks.

- Etiology/Risk Factors—due to infection with coxsackievirus A16
- Clinical diagnosis: Characteristic lesions—seen anywhere but especially on the oral mucosa, hands and feet; hand-foot-mouth disease. Rash on the buttocks is common.
- Coxsackievirus B also responsible for viral myocarditis
- Treatment is supportive care

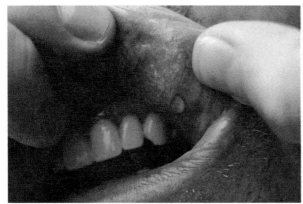

Copyright 2007 - Custom Medical Stock Photo.

Figure 22-4. Oral Ulcers of Hand-Foot-and-Mouth Disease

Adenovirus

A 12-year-old patient presents with fever, sore throat, and follicular conjunctivitis.

- Etiology/Risk Factors—DNA virus responsible for URIs in infants and children
- Clinical Presentation—Fever, pharyngitis, conjunctivitis, and diarrhea are common.
  - Less common features include pharyngoconjunctival fever, myocarditis, and intussusception.
- Diagnosis—serology, viral culture, or PCR, but not usually necessary
- Treatment—supportive

Poliovirus

- Etiology/Risk Factors—lives in gastrointestinal track
- Clinical Presentation—can cause URI symptoms
  - Paralytic polio
    - Asymmetric flaccid paralysis
- Prevent with vaccination

Acquired Immunodeficiency Syndrome (AIDS)

An 18-month-old has failure to thrive and developmental delay. The patient also has a history of recurrent ear infections, oral thrush, and chronic diarrhea. The patient on physical examination today is noted to have lymphadenopathy.

- Etiology/Risk Factors
  - Most are children born in developing countries; acquired at birth from an HIV-positive mother
  - Breast feeding in developing countries is an important route of transmission.
  - Pregnant females in United States and other developed countries are routinely screened for HIV infection in prenatal labs, unless the patient refuses.
    - Early treatment and prevention of neonatal infection through anti-retroviral therapy and preventive measures during delivery/postpartum period
- Clinical presentation
  - HIV-infected newborns: rapid onset of symptoms and AIDS in first few months of life
  - Initial symptoms may include
    - Lymphadenopathy
    - Hepatosplenomegaly
    - Failure to thrive
    - Chronic diarrhea
    - Interstitial pneumonia
    - Oral thrush
  - Children > adults: recurrent bacterial infections, chronic parotid swelling, lymphocytic interstitial pneumonitis, early progressive neurological deterioration
- Infections
  - **Recurrent bacterial infections with encapsulated organisms and other gram-positive and gram-negative organisms**
  - **Opportunistic infections**; most common is PCP (onset of fever, tachypnea, dyspnea, and marked hypoxemia)
  - **Mycobacterium avian-intracellulare complex**: disseminated disease in severely compromised
  - Oral candidiasis and other invasive fungal infections
  - Viral infections, especially herpes group
- Other problems
  - CNS disease
  - Cardiomyopathy
  - Enteropathy
  - Wasting syndrome, nephropathy
  - Many cutaneous manifestations
  - All hematologic manifestations, malignancies
- Diagnosis
  - **HIV-DNA by PCR**

- Maternal HIV IgG antibodies cross the placenta
  - Screen will be positive in **all** newborns up to age 18 months so need 2 of 3 ⊕ PCR for HIV in first month of life.
- In any **child >18 months of age**: test for infection through **IgG Ab by ELISA and then confirm with Western blot to establish the diagnosis.**
- Treatment—infants born to HIV-infected mothers
  - Mother should be on **perinatal triple anti-retroviral** therapy and then IV ZDV at start of labor until cord is clamped
  - Infant **should be started on ZDV (birth)** until neonatal disease is excluded
    - Also start **PCP prophylaxis (TMP-SMZ) at 1 month** until disease excluded
    - Follow CBC, platelets, CD4 and CD8 counts
    - With symptoms or evidence of immune dysfunction, should be treated with **antiretroviral therapy, regardless of age or viral load**
- Prognosis
  - Best single prognostic indicator is the **plasma viral load.**
  - Mortality higher with **CD4 count <15%**
  - Poor prognosis with persistent fever and/or thrush, serious bacterial infection (meningitis), hepatitis, persistent anemia, and/or thrombocytopenia (30% die by age 3)
  - Children with opportunistic infection, encephalopathy, or wasting syndrome have the worst prognosis (75% die by age <3)

HELMINTHIC DISEASES

Ascariasis

A child is brought to the physician's office because his mother found a "worm" while changing his diaper. He also has a chronic cough with pinkish sputum.

- Etiology/Pathogenesis—*Ascaris lumbricoides;* nematode (roundworm)
  - Most prevalent human helminth in the world
  - High prevalence in poor socioeconomic status countries, with use of human waste as fertilizer, and with geophagia (highest in preschool age)
  - Travels to the small intestines → releases larvae → migrates through venous circulation to lungs **and causes pulmonary ascariasis (Loeffler syndrome)** → through alveoli and bronchi to trachea and are swallowed mature in intestine to adult worms
- Clinical Presentation—most asymptomatic or mild
  - **Most common symptom is pulmonary disease—cough and blood-stained sputum**
  - Followed by obstructive intestinal or biliary tract disease
    - May have colicky abdominal pain or bile-stained emesis
  - CBC reveals **significant blood eosinophilia**
  - Can be identified on fecal smear
- Treatment—**albendazole,** mebendazole, or pyrantel pamoate

Note

Loeffler syndrome = pulmonary ascariasis plus hemoptysis

Hookworm

A 5-year-old girl is brought to the physician due to lack of appetite, abdominal pain, and diarrhea. On physical examination a yellow-green pallor is noted.

- Etiology/Risk Factors—*Ancylostoma duodenale* and *Necator americanus* are nematodes transmitted through warm, moist soil; usually in rural areas where human waste is used as fertilizer.
  - Penetrate **through the skin** (leads to intense pruritis at site of entry) or are ingested
  - Migration through veins to lungs and are swallowed → have teeth to attach to mucosa and can remain up to 5 years, where they mate and produce eggs
- Clinical Presentation—Morbidity from **blood loss**
  - **Iron deficiency anemia**
  - Hypoalbuminemia → edema, anasarca
  - Also, cough, colicky abdominal pain, anorexia, diarrhea
  - Physical growth retardation, cognitive and intellectual deficits
  - Green-yellow skin discoloration known as **chlorosis** and seen in chronic infection
  - Labs reveal significant **blood eosinophilia**.
  - Eggs can be identified on fecal smear.
- Treatment—**mebendazole or albendazole** is drug of choice; pyrantel pamoate an alternative
  - **Ferrous sulfate** if iron deficient

Note

Most parasites, ova, and cysts can be identified on fecal smear.

Enterobiasis

A mother brings her 4-year-old child to the physician with a history of always scratching her anus. The mother is embarrassed by this behavior. The child attends daycare and loves to play in the sandbox.

- Etiology—*Enterobius vermicularis* is the parasite implicated in pinworm infection.
  - Small, white, threadlike nematodes
  - Most common helminth in the United States
  - Primarily in institutional/family settings that include children; highest at age 5–14
  - Eggs are ingested from being carried on fingernails, clothing, bedding, or house dust; after ingestion, adult worms within 1–2 months
  - Inhabits cecum, appendix, ileus, and ascending colon; **female migration at night to deposit eggs on perianal region and perineum**
- Clinical Presentation—most common symptoms include **itching and restless sleep** and *no* eosinophilia
- Diagnosis—history and use of **adhesive cellophane tape** (tape test) **at night when child is asleep**
- Treatment—infected person and entire family receive **single oral dose of mebendazole and repeat in 2 weeks**

Adolescence 23

Learning Objectives

❏ Describe the epidemiology including morbidity and mortality of diseases of adolescence

❏ Answer questions related to adolescent sexuality and sexually transmitted diseases

❏ Describe the causes and treatments of acne

MORTALITY/MORBIDITY, SEXUALITY, AND STDS

A 14-year-old girl who has not yet achieved menarche presents to the physician with her concerned mother. The mother is afraid that her daughter is not "normal." On physical examination, the patient appears well nourished and is in the 50th percentile for height and weight. Her breast examination shows the areolar diameter to be enlarged, but there is no separation of contours. Her pubic hair is increased in amount and is curled but is not coarse in texture. The mother and her daughter wait anxiously for your opinion.

Introduction to Adolescence and Puberty

- Definition—period bridging childhood and adulthood
- Begins at age 11–12 years, ends at 18–21; includes puberty
- Physical and psychological/behavioral changes
    - Completes pubertal and somatic growth
    - Develops socially, cognitively and emotionally
        - Moves from concrete to abstract thinking
        - Establishes independent identity
        - Prepares for career
- All adolescents are at increased risk of mortality and morbidity.
    - Mortality
        - Accidents—especially MVAs
        - Suicide—boys are more successful
        - Homicide—more likely in blacks
        - Cancer—Hodgkin lymphoma, bone, CNS

- Morbidity
  - Unintended pregnancy
  - STDs
  - Smoking
  - Depression
  - Crime
- There are 3 stages of adolescence.
  - *Early (Age 10-14 years)*
    - Physical changes (puberty) including rapid growth, puberty including development of secondary sexual characteristics
    - Compare themselves to peers (develop body image and self-esteem)
    - Concrete thinkers and feel awkward
  - *Middle (Age 15-16 years)*
    - More independent and have a sense of **identity**
    - Mood swings are common.
    - Abstract thinking
    - Relationships are one-sided and narcissistic.
  - *Late (Age >17 years)*
    - Less self-centered
    - Relationships with individuals rather than groups
    - Contemplate future goals, plans, and careers
    - Idealistic; have a sense of right and wrong

Table 23-1. Tanner Stages of Development

	Female	Both	Male
Stage	Breast	Pubic hair	Genitalia
I	Preadolescent	None	Childhood size
II	Breast bud	Sparse, long, straight	Enlargement of scrotum/testes
III	Areolar diameter enlarges	Darker, curling, increased amount	Penis grows in length; testes continue to enlarge
IV	Secondary mound; separation of contours	Coarse, curly, adult type	Penis grows in length/breadth; scrotum darkens, testes enlarge
V	Mature female	Adult, extends to thighs	Adult shape/size

- Puberty
  - Variability in onset, duration
  - No variability in order of changes
  - Irreversible
  - Physical reflects hormonal

- Variants of development are normal and most cases only require **reassurance** from the physician to the patient and their family.
  - Breast asymmetry and gynecomastia often seen in males at Tanner stage 3
  - Irregular menses due to anovulatory cycles seen in females starting to menstruate

Sexually Transmitted Diseases

Gonorrhea

A 16-year-old girl presents to her physician because of fever, chills, pain, and swelling in the small joints of her hands, and a maculopapular rash on her upper and lower extremities.

- *Neisseria gonorrhoeae* usually infects mucosal membranes of the genitourinary tract and less commonly the oropharynx, rectum, and conjunctiva.
- Clinical presentation includes urethritis, cervicitis, and dysuria.
- Asymptomatic patients are at higher risk for dissemination, including fever, chills, and arthritis.
- Physical examination
  - Males present with dysuria and purulent penile discharge.
  - Females present with purulent vaginal discharge, cervicitis, abdominal pain, and/or dysuria.
  - Rectal gonorrhea may present with proctitis, rectal bleeding, anal discharge, and/or constipation.
- Tests
  - Culture from discharge
  - Blood cultures if dissemination is suspected
  - Gram stain may show intracellular diplococci.
- Check for other STDs, including **syphilis** and **HIV infection**.
- Treat with single-dose ceftriaxone or single-dose azithromycin; treat partners.
  - Alternatives include doxycycline for 7 days (**not** in children <9 years of age).

Note

Untreated GC/Chlamydia may result in PID and/or infertility (due to tubal scarring).

Chlamydia

A 16-year-old boy presents to the emergency center with a persistent penile discharge. The patient states that 1 week ago he saw his family physician for this same problem. At that time the physician gave him an IM shot of penicillin. However, the patient states that the discharge did not resolve with the penicillin therapy. He would like a second opinion.

- Cause of nongonococcal urethritis
- Intracellular obligate parasites
- Most common STD in developed countries
- Mucoid discharge (mostly females) or lymphogranuloma vernerum

- Tests
    - Nucleic acid amplification (**PCR, ELISA**)
    - Culture of infected tissue
- Treatment
    - Single-dose azithromycin or doxycycline for 7 days
    - Erythromycin if pregnant

Trichomonas

A 15-year-old presents to her physician because she has a yellow, foul-smelling vaginal discharge. On physical examination, she is noted to have a "strawberry cervix."

- *Trichomonas vaginalis* is a protozoa resulting in vaginitis
- Girls with multiple sexual partners (although this is the case in all STDs) are at high risk.
- Frothy, foul-smelling vaginal discharge; males asymptomatic
- "Strawberry cervix" due to hemorrhages in the mucosa
- Wet prep shows motile protozoans in females
- In males, examine urine sediment after prostatic massage
- Treat with metronidazole

Herpes

A 17-year-old, sexually active boy presents to the physician because of painful ulcerations on his glans penis and on the shaft of his penis. He has multiple sexual partners and does not use condoms. Fever and inguinal adenopathy are also present.

- HSV 1: nongenital infections of mouth, eye, and lips most common
- HSV 2: genital, neonatal, oral
    - Cervix primary site in girls; penis in boys
    - Tzanck prep—giant multinuclear cells
    - ELISA testing
- Treat with acyclovir, valacyclovir, famciclovir

Table 23-2. Distinguishing Features of Vaginal Discharge

Feature	Bacterial vaginosis	Trichomoniasis	Candida	Chlamydia/gonorrhea
Discharge	Profuse, malodorous, "fishy"	Gray-green, frothy	Cottage cheese	Purulent
Wet prep	Clue cells, "whiff test" with KOH	Motile Trichomonads	Hyphae seen with KOH prep	WBCs
pH	>4.5	>5	<4.5	—
STD	No	Yes	No	Yes

ACNE

A mother brings her 15-year-old daughter to the dermatologist because she has developed pimples. The mother says that her daughter's face "breaks out" because she drinks soda pop. The daughter is argumentative about this but admits that she does drink soda pop every day at lunch. The mother would like you to tell her daughter to stop drinking soda pop. On physical examination, the patient has open and closed comedones and pimples on her forehead, nose, and cheeks.

- Pathogenesis
  - Due to the bacteria—*Propionibacterium acnes*, which forms free fatty acids within the sebaceous follicle
  - Abnormal keratinization of follicular epithelium and impaction of keratinized cells in sebaceous follicles
  - Increased sebum production—At puberty, significant increase in sebum from increased **adrenal androgens** (mostly DHEAS with some role of testosterone and estrogen)
  - Inflammation from lysosomal enzymes, which phagocytose bacteria
- Description
  - **Open comedone** = blackhead
  - **Closed comedone** = whitehead (more commonly becomes inflammatory)
  - If comedones rupture, inflammatory lesion and inflammatory contents spill into adjacent dermis; if close to the surface, forms a **papule or pustule**; deeper forms a **nodule**
  - With suppuration → giant-cell reaction to keratin and hair; forms **nodulocystic lesion**
- Treatment must be individualized.
  - Cleansing of skin with mild soap
  - Topical therapy used for treatment of comedones and papulopustular acne
    - **Benzoyl peroxide**
    - **Tretinoin (Retin-A): single most effective agent for comedonal acne**
    - **Adapalene** (Differen gel)

- - Topical antibiotics: **erythromycin or clindamycin**
  - Allow 4–8 weeks to assess effect of above agents
- Systemic treatment is indicated in those who do not respond to topical agents.
  - Antibiotics: especially **tetracycline,** minocycline, doxycycline, erythromycin, clindamycin
  - **Isotretinoin: for moderate to severe nodulocystic disease.** Very **teratogenic**; contraindicated in pregnancy. Other major side effect is increased **triglycerides and cholesterol**: rule out liver disease prior to start and check triglycerides 4 weeks after starting treatment
  - **A trial of hormonal therapy can be used in those who are not candidates for isotretinoin.**
- Corticosteroid injections may be used to aid in healing painful nodulocystic lesions.
- Dermabrasion may help decrease visible scarring.

Note

Isotretinoin is very **teratogenic** and contraindicated in pregnancy.

Index

H

I